Horse
Healthcare

For Chrissie

Horse Healthcare

A Manual for Animal Health Workers and Owners

David Hadrill

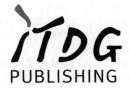

ITDG
PUBLISHING

Published by ITDG Publishing
103–105 Southampton Row, London WC1B 4HL, UK
www.itdgpublishing.org.uk

© David Hadrill 2002
First published in 2002

ISBN 1 85339 486 6

Main illustrator: Chris Tomlin
Cartoonist: Jawed Iqbal
Other drawings by David Hadrill, Hannah Lawson,
Neil Harvey and Christine Gent

ITDG Publishing is the publishing arm of the Intermediate Technology Development Group.
Our mission is to build the skills and capacity of people in developing countries through the
dissemination of information in all forms, enabling them to improve the quality of their lives
and that of future generations.

Disclaimer

This book is intended to assist those working in situations where resources and veterinary services
are limited or unavailable. The author and publisher assume no responsibility for and make no warranty
with respect to the results of using the techniques, diagnoses and treatments described in this book.
The author and publisher accept no liability whatsoever for any damage or loss resulting from use of
or reliance on any information contained in this book.

Since this book will enjoy wide distribution, the veterinary procedures and medicines recommended here
do not and cannot comply with all the laws of each sovereign country. Before performing any procedure,
giving veterinary advice or treating any animal with drugs the reader is responsible for familiarizing
himself or herself with the local laws and regulations that apply to the practice of veterinary medicine and
drug use and for strict adherence to those laws.

This book is not intended to substitute for the complete prescribing information prepared by each
manufacturer for each drug. The data sheet and directions for use and precautions for every drug product
should be read, understood and followed before any drug is administered or prescribed.

Designed and typeset by Technical Art Services, Stanstead Abbotts, Hertfordshire, England
Printed in Great Britain

Contents

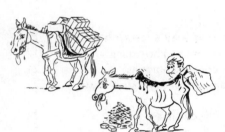

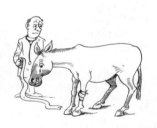

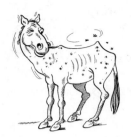

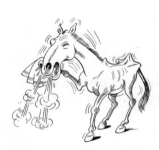

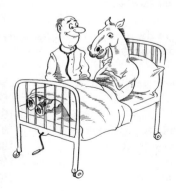

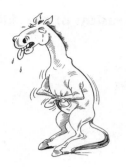

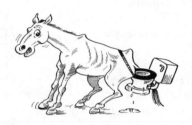

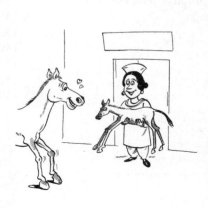

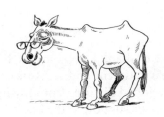

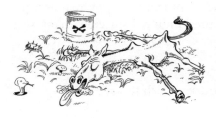

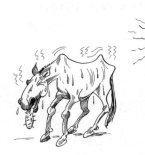

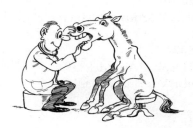

Acknowledgements

Many people helped make this book. I would particularly like to thank P.J.N. Pinsent, BVSc, FRCVS. He taught me horse medicine when I was a veterinary student and scrutinized the manuscript. I am grateful to all the artists who patiently developed pictures from my ideas, especially Chris Tomlin, MA (RCA). Brooke Hospital for Animals supported the book's production in many ways, financial and technical. Special thanks are due to Rick Butson, BVSc, Cert VA, Cert ES (Orth), Dip ECVS, MRCVS and to Joy Pritchard, BVM&S, MRCVS.

Between them, the people listed below have made contributions to the text, posed for photographs or provided other reference for the illustrator, and commented on the manuscript. Thomas Burch, RSS did all of these! Others helped to secure funding. I sincerely thank you all for your help and advice.

J.O.S. Belgrave	Director, Vetstream plc
Roy Brown	Horseman and Restaurateur, Bardsley's Fish Restaurant, Brighton, UK
Thomas Burch	Farrier to the Metropolitan Police, London
Rick Butson	BHA Overseas Development Director
Martyn Edelsten	Senior Lecturer, Centre for Tropical Veterinary Medicine, University of Edinburgh
BHA Egypt	Dr Emad and staff at the Luxor Clinic
Claire Goddings	Head Nurse, Equine Veterinary Hospital, Arundel, UK
Archie Hunter	Senior Lecturer, Centre for Tropical Veterinary Medicine, University of Edinburgh
BHA India	Brig Rappai and BHA Delhi staff
BHA Jordan	Petra Clinic staff and former Veterinary Officers, Bassam Naser and Ismail Muraweh
Patrick Krause	Chief Executive, VETAID
Mark Lainchbury	Former BHA Director of Veterinary Services
Tony Luckins	Honorary Fellow, Centre for Tropical Veterinary Medicine, University of Edinburgh
Will Matthews	Veterinarian, Equine Veterinary Hospital, Arundel, UK
BHA Pakistan	BHA Lahore and Peshawar staff
Brian Patterson	Veterinarian, Equine Veterinary Hospital, Arundel, UK
Anne Pearson	Senior Reseach Fellow, Centre for Tropical Veterinary Medicine, University of Edinburgh
Jim Pinsent	Formerly Senior Lecturer, School of Veterinary Science, University of Bristol
Joy Pritchard	BHA Veterinary Advisor
Christine Purdy	Former BHA Chief Executive
Col. Manzoor Waheed	Chief Veterinary Officer, BHA Pakistan
Alan Walker	Senior Lecturer, Royal (Dick) School of Veterinary Studies, University of Edinburgh

David Hadrill

Introduction

How to find what you want in the book

1. Contents list

To find the section you want, look at the *Contents* at the beginning of the book. This gives the chapter headings and sub-headings. For example, if you want to know how to treat an animal for worms, in the *Contents* you will find Chapter 13, *Diarrhoea, worms and other parasites living inside the body*. As sub-headings, you will see *Red-worm disease, Large roundworms (ascarid worms)* and *Tapeworms*. Read these sections to decide which kinds of worms you may need to treat and how to treat them.

2. Index

At the back of the book, there is an *Index*. For each subject listed, the page number of the main reference is given in **bold typeface**.

3. Medicine lists

At the back of the book before the index, there are lists of the medicines mentioned in the book. These give a summary of what the medicines are used for and how to give them.

When to get more help

It is not recommended that untrained people attempt some of the techniques described in the book, for example using a stomach tube. These techniques are indicated with the warning triangle sign.

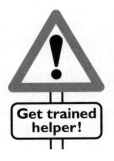

This symbol is used in the book to show when you may need more help

About this book

This book has been written to guide readers on the appropriate action to take when caring for a sick horse, donkey or mule, in situations where they do not have professional advice. The book explains how to provide veterinary care and how to prevent many common illnesses.

The book is not intended to replace the role of the veterinary profession where an adequate animal health service exists. In poorer countries, however, owners may have no alternative but to treat their sick animals with whatever resources and advice are available locally. It is hoped that this book will help reduce animal suffering in these situations, where access to veterinary services is limited.

In order that the book is useful to more people, complicated or technical language has been avoided where possible. Also, there are many pictures to help make the text easier to understand.

Parts of the book may be copied freely, provided the conditions stated at the front of the book are followed. BHA and the author would be interested to see a copy of any training material made using material from this book. Please send it to:

David Hadrill
c/o Brooke Hospital for Animals
21 Panton Street
London SW1Y 4DR
UK

Please send suggestions for improvements to this book to David Hadrill at the same address.

How to tie, restrain and transport horses and donkeys

1.1 How to tie useful knots

Quick-release knots

Horses should be tied using a quick-release knot. Then, if the animal goes down, the knot can be undone quickly, reducing the risk of strangling or injury.

QUICK-RELEASE KNOT (1)

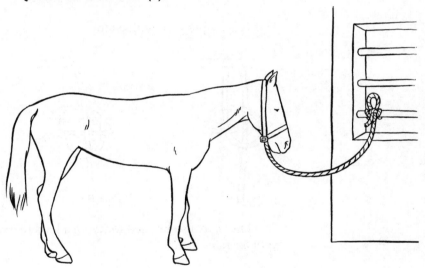

To tie this knot, put a loop through a loop through a loop, and pull tight.

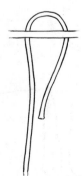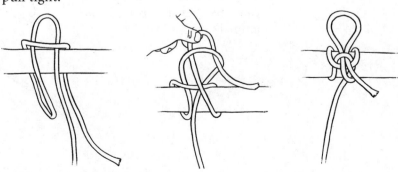

Pull the short end to untie quickly.

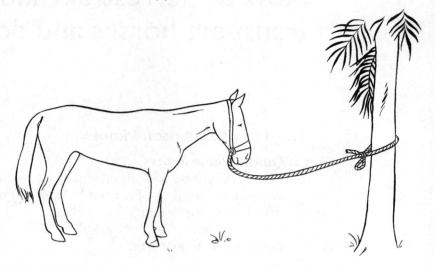

This is a simple knot with a loop.

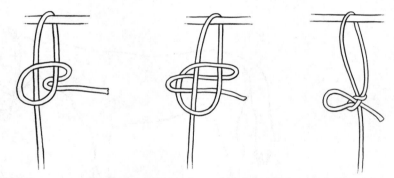

This knot can also be used for tying a load to a horse, see the section *Knot for tying loads*.

Bowline

The bowline knot is a fixed loop. It cannot pull tight. It can be used around an animal's neck.

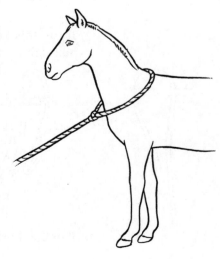

HOW TO MAKE A BOWLINE KNOT

1 Take a length of rope and make a loop in it by laying the shorter end over the long end.

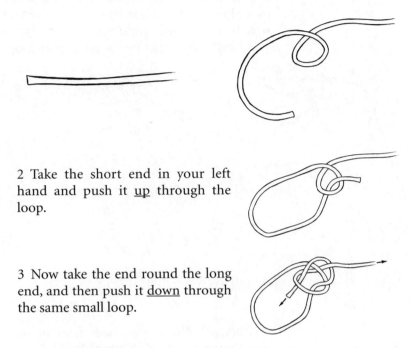

2 Take the short end in your left hand and push it <u>up</u> through the loop.

3 Now take the end round the long end, and then push it <u>down</u> through the same small loop.

4 Pull the knot tight and check that you have tied a loop big enough to go over the horse's head without being tight around its neck.

Knot for tying loads

Use a quick-release knot, in case you need to take the load off the animal quickly, for example, if it falls. Quick-release knot (2) described above can be used to tie the rope to a loop.

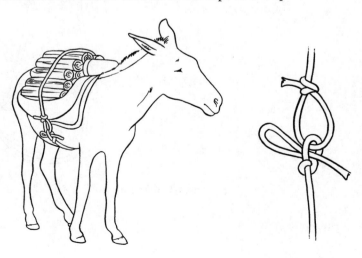

1.2   How to restrain horses and donkeys

Halter

If a horse or donkey's head is restrained, it can be led or held for procedures such as injections. A halter can be made from a piece of sisal or cotton rope. Avoid using nylon rope against the skin.

A simple slip halter can be made with loops.

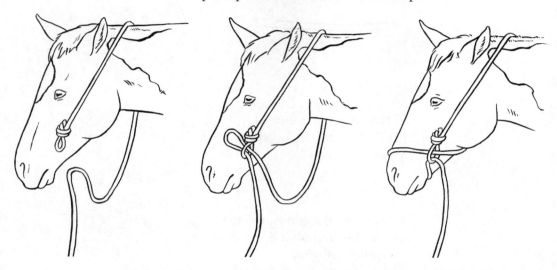

A better halter can be made from about 5 metres of rope. The rope should be about 15 mm wide. Make a small loop at one end of the rope and another loop about 30 cm along. Then thread the end through the loops as shown in the next pictures.

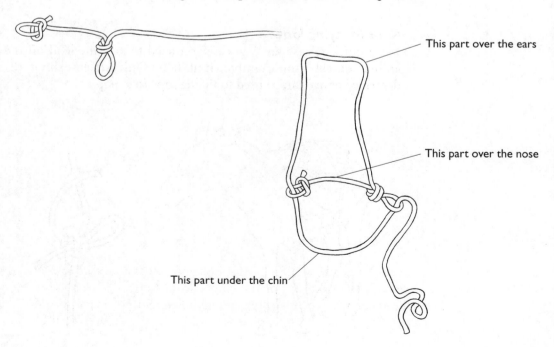

This part over the ears

This part over the nose

This part under the chin

The halter on the animal

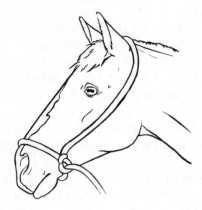

Make sure that the fixed piece of rope between the two loops is above the nose. A small knot made with the free end of the rope stops the halter becoming too tight across the head.

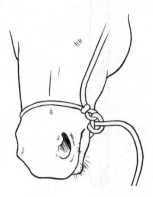

Head collar
Some horses learn to slip halters off over the ears. A head collar is better.

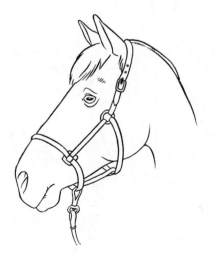

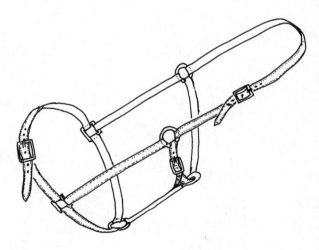

Head collars are suitable for donkeys too, but should have buckles to adjust the size of the straps around the nose. This way the head collar can be made big enough to go around a donkey's nose.

Twitch

The twitch is useful to restrain a horse before a painful procedure, to examine it or give it treatment. A horse will normally stand still when the twitch has been put on.

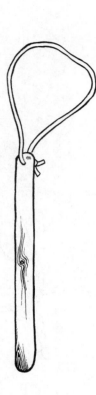

It is known that a twitch placed correctly on the nose causes the release of natural pain-killing substances in the horse's body. Twitches are not as useful for donkeys, which seem to be frightened by them.

A twitch can be made from a wooden pole or long axe handle with a hole in the end. A rope loop about 50 cm long is tied through the hole.

To put the twitch on the upper lip, first put three fingers and thumb through the loop. If you hold the lip with three fingers like this, the loop does not get caught over your hand when you start to tighten it.

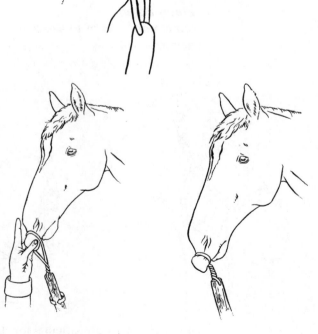

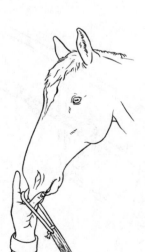

Hold the lip, slip on the loop and twist the pole.

- Do not tighten the twitch more than necessary to restrain the horse.

- Do not keep a twitch tight for more than 10 minutes.
- Never put a twitch on the ear. It is cruel and can damage the ear.
- Do not put a twitch on the lower jaw either.

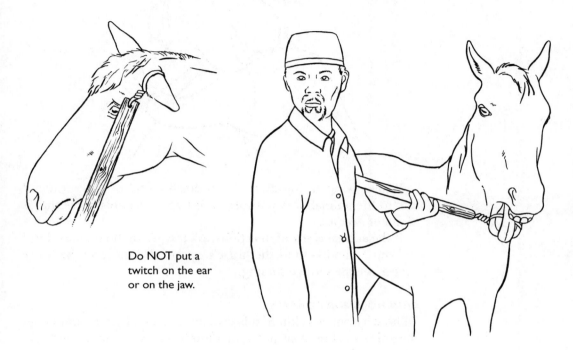

Do NOT put a
twitch on the ear
or on the jaw.

Mild restraint without a twitch

Although you must never put a twitch on to an ear, you can steady
the head by holding an ear.

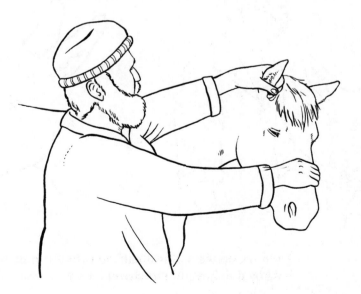

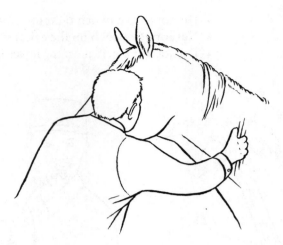

While giving an injection, if you pinch a fold of neck skin and talk to the animal, it is possible to distract a nervous horse that is afraid of needles.

If the animal is shy of injections, ask the person holding the head to keep a hand behind the horse's eye on that side, so the horse cannot see the syringe coming.

CHIN HOLD FOR DONKEYS

To hold a donkey's chin in this way, put the flat of your hand under the animal's chin, then put your thumb across its mouth and grip with your fingers.

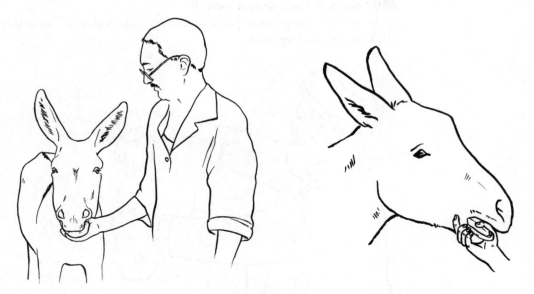

For most donkeys, this is sufficient, but if more restraint is needed, hold by the chin and the base of an ear.

BLINDFOLDING

Covering a horse's eyes with a towel or similar cloth will often make it stand quietly. In a confined space the horse may back away at first and become frightened if it collides with things. Blindfolding is more useful in a field.

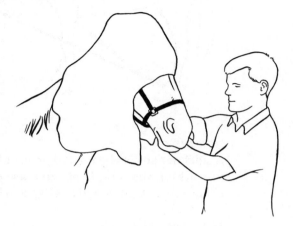

How to prevent kicking

LIFT UP A FRONT LEG

This technique helps to prevent kicking from a back leg. It can help to keep the hind legs still so work can be done on them. Pick up the front leg on the same side as the back leg on which you are working.

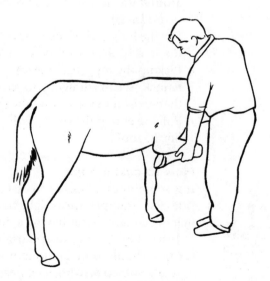

Call vet!

It is easier if two people restrain the horse. One person keeps the head still, while the other holds up the front leg.

This method is not suitable for a very nervous horse. If possible, get a vet to sedate a very difficult animal with an injection. Do not sedate if the animal has to go back to work immediately afterwards.

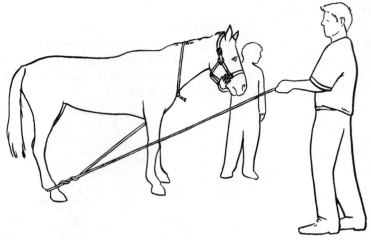

SIDELINE

A sideline can also be used to prevent kicking or to lift up a hind leg to work on the foot. If possible use cotton rope, not nylon rope. Cotton rope is softer and less likely to burn the skin.

How to put on a sideline
- Wrap a strip of old cloth or bandage around the leg below the fetlock, if it can be done safely without danger of being kicked. This will prevent the sideline rope from injuring the skin. Have a front leg lifted up while you do it.
- For the loop that goes round the neck, pass the end of the rope around the neck and tie a bowline knot (see the section *How to tie useful knots*).
- Lay the long end of the rope on the ground and walk the animal forward so the rope is between its hind legs.
- Pick up the rope, pass the long end around the hind leg at the fetlock (see the drawing on page 51 for position of the fetlock), then twist it twice around the rope from the neck.
- Pull the end of the rope gently to stop the animal kicking, or to lift the foot.

How to cast a horse

It is sometimes necessary to cast an animal, that is, make it lie on its side. For example, this might be done to avoid being kicked when helping a mare that is having a difficult birth.

Instead of casting, veterinarians usually give a sedative injection. Casting should only be done if a vet is not available to sedate the animal. Someone who is experienced in casting should lead the team of helpers.

What you need
- At least five people: one to hold the head and two to pull each rope.
- A strong halter or head collar on the horse.

- A long piece of rope, 15 metres long and 1.0–1.5 cm thick, to cast the animal. Cotton rope is best, as it does not rub the skin as much as rope made of other materials.
- A shorter piece of rope about 3 metres long, to go around the chest.
- Bandages for the legs.

Before you start
- Find a place with soft ground without rocks or stones, which could injure the animal when it goes down.
- If possible, do not let the animal eat for 12 hours before so its guts are not full when it is cast.
- Bandage the lower parts of all four legs to prevent ropes from injuring the skin.
- Decide who is in charge. This person will give the instruction to pull the ropes when everything is ready.
- To reduce confusion, tell the other people that they should all keep quiet.
- Check that everyone knows what they have to do.

How to do it
- Make sure that the person who will hold the head is experienced and knows what he/she has to do. The person at the head must be told not to let go of the head. This person must also be told not to let the horse bend its neck as it goes down (or the horse's neck or back may be injured).
- Lay the rope on the ground, double.

- Make a loop with a figure-of-eight knot. This kind of knot is flat against the animal's breast.

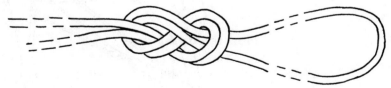

- Coil up each end of rope.
- Place the loop over the head.
- Tie the shorter length of rope around the chest and attach it to the loop around the neck (this is to stop the neck loop slipping forward if the animal struggles).
- If the horse is nervous, get someone to hold up a front leg. See above, *How to prevent kicking*.
- Pass the coiled ends of rope between the front legs, backwards

and round over the hocks of the back legs. If these ropes are over the hocks at this stage, even if the horse kicks, the ropes will stay around the legs.

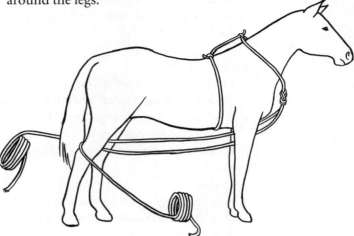

- Bring the coiled ends of rope forwards under the first part of rope.
- Pass these ends through the neck loop.
- Two people hold the end of one rope well in front of the animal.
- Two other people hold the end of the other rope well behind the animal.
- Let the loops of rope around the back legs slip down so they are just above the hooves.

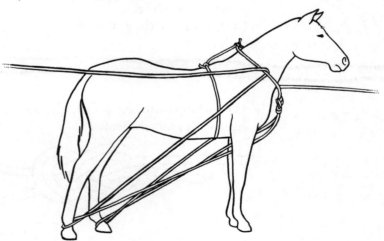

- The person in charge gives the order 'Pull!'
- The person on the head makes the horse move backwards.
- The pairs of people pull their ropes and the animal goes into a sitting position.
- The person on the head must stop the animal from bending its neck, or it may injure its neck or back.
- As soon as the animal is sitting, it can be turned over on to its side.

- The upper back leg is now pulled up to the shoulder and tied with two or three loops (half hitches) just above the hoof with the end of the rope on that side.
- Now the front foot is tied in the same way beside the back foot.
- The animal is turned over and the other back and front legs are tied in the same way.
- The person in charge of the head keeps control of it all the time that the horse is cast.

How to cast a donkey

As for casting a horse:

- Make sure the donkey is wearing a head collar or halter.
- Have a reliable person control the head.
- Find a suitable area of soft ground.

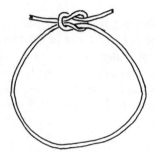 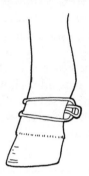 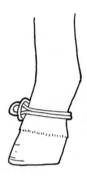

- Make four rope loops to make four hobbles.
- Put the hobbles around the legs.
- Thread a piece of rope through all the hobbles and tie it to one as shown in the picture.

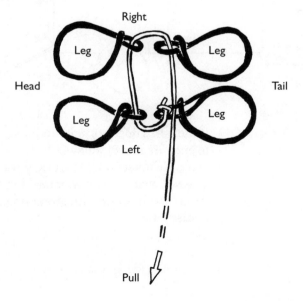

- When the rope is pulled, the donkey will go down on to its right side.
- Tie the feet together.
- Keep control of the head until the feet are untied and the animal is allowed to stand.

1.3 How to transport animals

Loading into a truck

It can be difficult to persuade an animal to walk into a truck if it is not trained for this. This advice can make it easier:

- Bring the vehicle to the animal. Do not make an injured animal walk more than absolutely necessary.
- Park the truck with one side along a wall so the animal cannot escape round that side.
- One person should lead the horse, holding the halter rope.
- Two other people pass a rope around the back end of the horse. One stands each side of the animal and takes the end of the rope on their own side. They pull steadily forward. (With only one person at the side of the horse, a rope can be tied to something at the side of the truck, looped around the back end of the horse and pulled.)

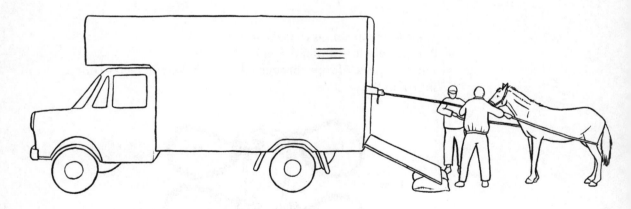

- If the horse does not want to move, use a broom behind the horse to encourage it to walk in.
- Once the horse is in the truck, reward it with some tasty food. This will help make it more willing to walk in next time.
- Secure the head by tying the animal's head collar using a quick-release knot.

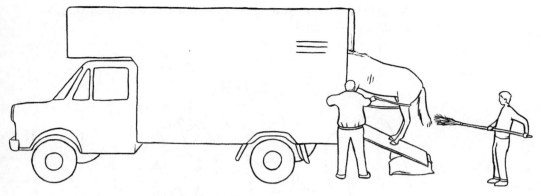

Transporting

- Always drive at a sensible speed, even if it seems to be an emergency.
- If a hind leg is injured, have the animal face the direction of travel. Then when the vehicle slows it can take the weight on its front legs during braking.
- If a front leg is injured, turn the animal so it looks back if possible. Then it can take the forces on its back legs when the vehicle is braking.
- Partitions allow the animal to lean sideways. Use partitions to allow the animal only a little sideways movement.

Lifting and moving an injured or sick animal

A very, very weak horse on the ground might need help to stand up. As a horse gets up front end first, help it stand up with a pole under its chest just behind the front legs. One person lifts each end of the pole.

Two men can carry a donkey. They reach under the donkey's belly and grasp each other's arms.

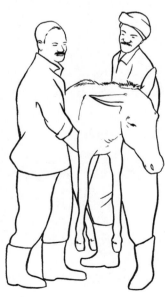

A horse that is too weak to stand can be rolled on to strong sacking and dragged along.

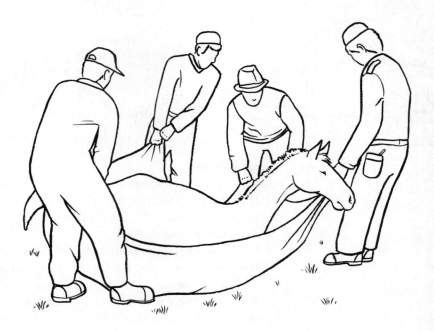

If a horse or donkey is too weak to stand and is suffering, consider euthanasia. After some time, the muscles become damaged and the animal is unlikely ever to stand. A horse is unlikely to stand again if it has been down for more than three days, a donkey if it has been down for more than five days.

2 How to check signs of a horse or donkey's health

2.1 Temperature, heart rate and breathing

The tables below show, for different animals, the normal temperatures, pulse (heart rate) and number of breaths taken per minute for an animal at rest. The number of heart beats and breaths per minute increases after exercise. Count these when the animal is rested.

The mean or average values are in bold type, for example, 37.7. The ranges found in normal animals are in brackets, for example, (37.5–38.0).

Normal temperature, heart rate and breathing for donkeys

	Body temperature of healthy animals (°C)	Normal pulse rate (heart beats per minute)	Normal number of breaths per minute
Young donkey	37.6 (37.1–38.1)	60 (50–70)	28 (20–40)
Adult donkey	37.0 (36.5–37.5)	45 (35–55)	20 (15–35)

Normal temperature, heart rate and breathing for horses

	Body temperature of healthy animals (°C)	Normal pulse rate (heart beats per minute)	Normal number of breaths per minute
Foal, 1 week old	38.5 (38.0–39.0)	100 (80–120)	15 (14–16)
Pony	37.7 (37.5–38.0)	40 (35–45)	14 (12–15)
Horse	37.7 (37.5–38.0)	36 (30–40)	13 (12–15)

In cool climates, it is not normal for a horse or pony to take more than 20 breaths per minute, but in hot countries there may be 30 breaths per minute.

How to read a thermometer

Take the thermometer out of its case and hold it between the thumb and forefinger. Roll it until you can see a broad silver band of mercury.

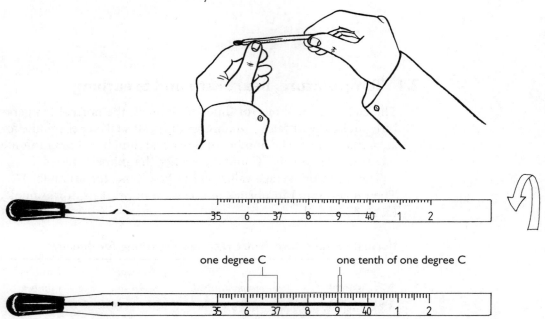

one degree C   one tenth of one degree C

Look at the scale on the thermometer. Can you recognize the marks for a whole degree and those for 0.1 (one tenth) of a degree?

How to take the temperature

- If the reading is not below 36°C, shake the mercury down to the bulb. Use flicking motions, taking care not to hit the thermometer on anything.

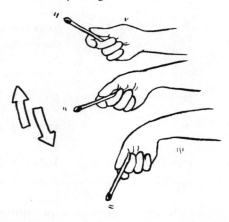

- Put a halter or head collar on the horse or donkey and have an assistant hold the head.

- Wet the thermometer with cold water or put some petroleum jelly (Vaseline) on the end to make it more slippery.
- Stand beside the horse or donkey, just in front of its back leg, with your body against the animal's body. Horses do not usually kick forward, so this is safer than standing behind the animal. If the horse does not stand quietly, an assistant should hold up a front leg (see the section *How to restrain horses and donkeys*).

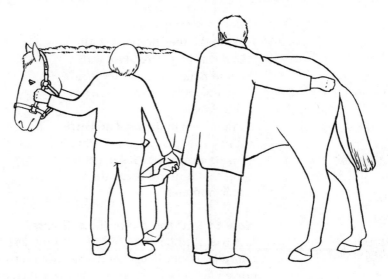

- Hold the tail away from the anus, and put the bulb of the thermometer gently into the centre of the anus.

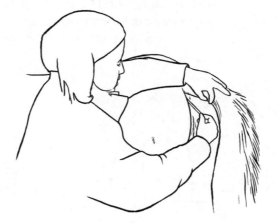

- If the animal tightly closes its anal ring so the thermometer will not go in easily, remove the thermometer until the muscles of the ring relax and then put it in again.
- Move the thermometer so the bulb is against the side of the rectum (the temperature at the centre of a ball of dung may be less than the body temperature). Keep hold of the end of the thermometer.

- Wait 60 seconds (or longer if the instructions on your thermometer tell you that longer is required).
- Remove the thermometer and clean it. Wipe it on the animal's hair, or on some tissue paper, or on cotton wool.
- Read the temperature.
- Wash the thermometer with *cold* running water. Hot water could make the mercury inside expand so much that it breaks the glass.
- Put it back in its case and keep it in a cool place. Do not leave it inside a car where it can get so hot that it might break the thermometer.

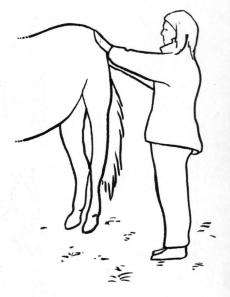

How to find the pulse (heart) rate

It is useful to be able to find out how fast the heart is beating. For example, it can help you decide whether colic is serious. An adult horse's heart beats more slowly than ours, especially when the horse is fit.

It takes practice to find the pulse. There are several places where it can be felt. Using a watch with a second hand, count how many beats can be felt in a minute.

Feel for it under the bone (mandible) at the side of the face.

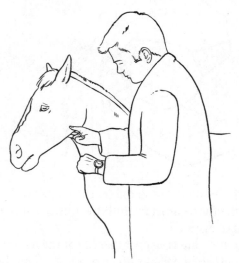

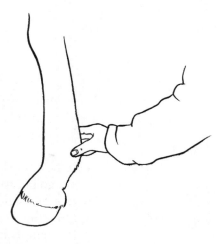

Or feel for it behind the fetlock joint.

Or feel for it just above the hoof on the inside of the leg. It is useful to practise finding the pulse here because, if the horse has laminitis, this pulse will feel stronger. If you know what the pulse normally feels like here, it will help you recognize when it is different.

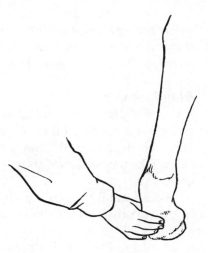

Or listen to the heart beat with your ear pressed on the animal's chest, just behind its elbow.

2.2 How to check mucous membranes

The mucous membranes include the inside of the eyelids, the gums and the inside of the lips of the mare's vulva. The colour of the normally pink skin inside the eyelids can change and can be a sign indicating some diseases.

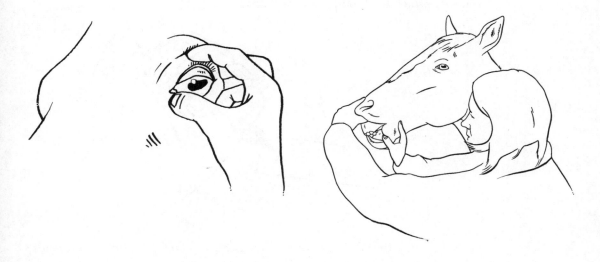

2.3 How to collect samples for laboratory tests

Dung sample

Dung samples are needed to check for worm eggs. Fresh samples are needed.

Watch an animal until it passes dung. Turn a clean polythene bag inside out and put it on your hand like a glove, pick up a pellet of dung (about 50 g), turn the bag out over the sample and tie it. If the sample will not be examined promptly, keep it in a refrigerator.

Blood sample

Use a new disposable syringe and needle or a sterilized, re-usable syringe and needle. Follow the method in *Injection into the jugular vein (intravenous or 'IV' injection)* in the section *How to give injections*. Take the needle off the syringe, and squirt the blood into the collection bottle.

The laboratory which is going to do tests on the sample should be able to provide a suitable small bottle for the blood.

- If the laboratory needs serum (the clear, yellowish fluid left after blood has clotted) for tests, it will provide a bottle without any chemical to stop clotting. In this case, allow the bottle to stand in a warm place for an hour so the blood clots.
- If the laboratory needs unclotted blood, fill the special bottle to the right line. Then, roll the bottle in your hands a few times so that the blood mixes with the chemical that stops it clotting.

Blood smear

To make a blood smear you need perfectly clean glass microscope slides. Place a drop of blood near the end of one of the slides on which the blood smear will be made.

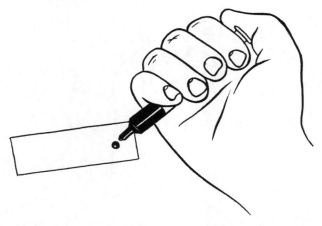

Bring the edge of another slide back to it so the blood drop spreads sideways. Keeping the slides in contact spread the blood along.

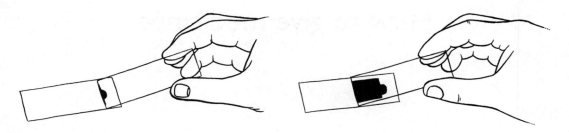

If the drop of blood was neither too big nor too small, there should be a thin film of blood smeared along the slide. The smear should become thinner and run out of blood before the end of the slide.

Skin scraping

Skin scrapings can be used to detect small parasites of the skin (see the chapter *Diseases and parasites of the skin*). A scraping is usually taken from thickened, diseased skin.

To make a skin scraping, you need a sharp blade, such as a disposable scalpel blade or a razor blade. Some liquid paraffin (<u>not</u> the kerosene type of paraffin used for fuel) is useful to soften the skin. A laboratory may be able to provide 10% potassium hydroxide solution as an alternative liquid for softening the skin.

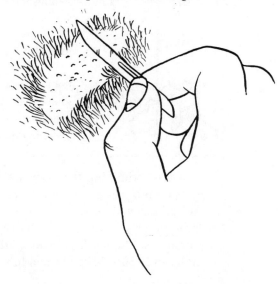

- With a piece of cotton wool wetted with either liquid paraffin or potassium hydroxide solution, moisten an area of skin about 3 cm wide.
- Scrape the area with the edge of the blade so that surface skin collects on it.
- Put the blade and sample in a bottle or wrap it in tinfoil to take for examining with a microscope.

3 How to give medicines

3.1 How to estimate body weight

It is important to know an animal's approximate body weight in order to work out how much medicine to give it. (The dose is usually worked out as the amount per kilogram of body weight. Thus, a 200 kg animal would need twice as much medicine as a 100 kg animal.)

Approximate body weights of horses, mules and donkeys

	Type of animal	Body weight
	Adult horse	400–500 kg
	Adult pony	300–400 kg
	Yearling horse	200–300 kg
	Newborn foal (of 450 kg mare)	40–50 kg
	Adult mule	350–450 kg
	Adult male donkey	300 kg
	Adult female donkey	200–250 kg
	Young donkey	100–150 kg
	Newborn donkey foal	30 kg

When estimating the body weight of a particular animal, think whether it is a larger or smaller breed, or if the animal is fat or thin, and adjust your estimate up or down. For example, in Pakistan some experts consider that the typical body weight of their native animals is 250–350 kg for an adult horse, 250–350 kg for an adult mule, and 150–250 kg for an adult donkey.

3.2 How to work out the amount of medicine to give

- Check the dose of the medicine, usually written on the container or on a piece of paper supplied with the bottle.
- Estimate the weight of the animal (see the section above, *How to estimate body weight*).
- Work out the amount to give (see examples opposite).

Example 1

A medicine has 5 ml/100 kg written on the packaging. This means 5 ml of medicine for each 100 kg body weight of animal.

If the animal weighs less than 100 kg, you need to inject less. If it weighs more, you need to inject more.

In this example, here are the amounts to give of a medicine with the dose of 5 ml/100 kg:

If the animal weighs 50 kg, inject 2.5 ml.
If the animal weighs 200 kg, inject 10 ml.
If the animal weighs 400 kg, inject 20 ml.
(If the animal weighs x kg, give x/100 × 5 ml).

Example 2

Another medicine is to be given at a dose of 5 mg/kg. This means 5 mg of medicine for each kg of body weight of animal. The medicine package says that each ml contains 100 mg of the drug.

In this example:

If the animal weighs 200 kg it needs 200 × 5 = 1000 mg of drug. As 1 ml contains 100 mg, 10 ml contains 1000 mg. Therefore, give 10 ml.

If the animal weighs 400 kg it needs 400 × 5 = 2000 mg of drug. As 1 ml contains 100 mg, 20 ml contains 2000 mg. Therefore, give 20 ml.

3.3 How to give injections

Syringes and needles
Some syringes are marked cc and some with ml. Cubic centimetres (cc) and millilitres (ml) are the same.

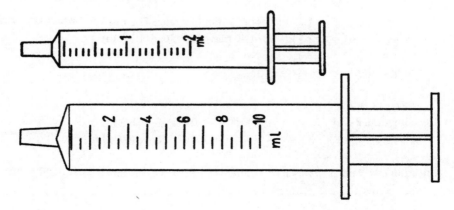

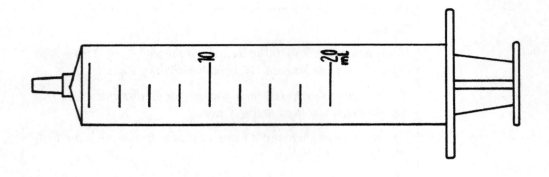

Read the amount here

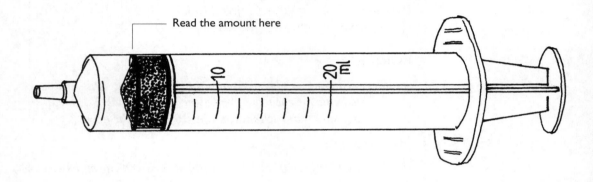

Recommended needle sizes for horses and donkeys

Type of injection	Length of needle	Width of needle	Needle actual size
Injection into muscle			
Adult horse or donkey	1.5 inches or 40 mm	20 gauge (0.9 mm)	
	or 1.5 inches or 40 mm	19 gauge (1.1 mm)	
	or 1 inch or 25 mm	19 gauge (1.1 mm)	
Thin, adult donkey	1 inch or 25 mm	20 gauge (0.9 mm)	
Foal	1 inch or 25 mm	21 gauge (0.8 mm)	
Large horse and thick substance to be injected (e.g. long-acting penicillin)	1.25 inches or 32 mm or 1.5 inches or 40 mm	18 gauge (1.2 mm) 18 gauge (1.2 mm)	
Injection under skin	1 inch or 25 mm	21 gauge (0.8 mm) or 23 gauge (0.6 mm)	
Injection into vein	1 inch or 25 mm	21 gauge (0.8 mm)	

How to handle a syringe and needle

Needles and the medicine inside a syringe go into the body. They have to be perfectly clean or the injection site can get infected. Therefore, the syringe and needle must be either disposable equipment taken from new wrapping, or sterilized by boiling for 10 minutes.

How to attach a needle to a syringe

Attach a disposable needle to a syringe by holding the needle cover, like this.

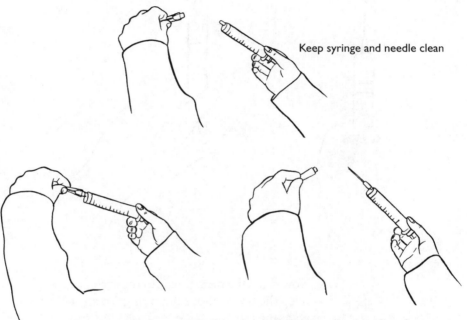

Keep syringe and needle clean

Never touch the metal, thin part of the needle (or dirt from your fingers may go into the animal). If you drop the needle, do not use it. Use a new one (or a re-usable one that has been sterilized).

How to load a syringe

- Be sure the needle is firmly attached.
- Draw some air into the syringe by pulling back the plunger.

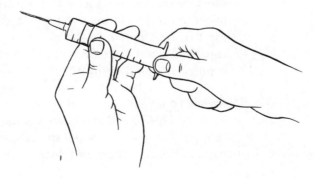

- Turn the bottle of medicine upside-down, insert the needle through the centre of the rubber stopper and slowly inject air into the bottle.

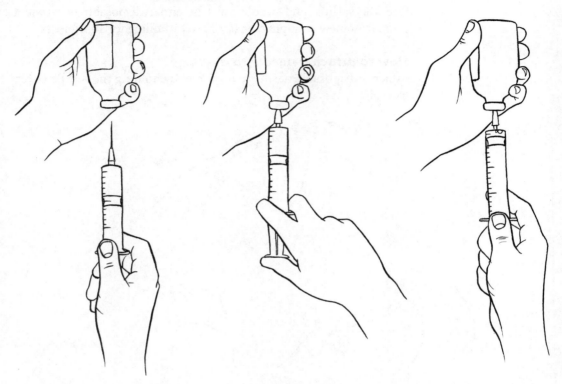

- Now draw the medicine into the syringe.
- Keep the bottle above the syringe so any air bubbles in the syringe go to the top.
- Push the plunger carefully so the air comes out.
- Now see if the right amount is in the syringe (the top of the plunger should be on the line for the proper dose).
- Withdraw more medicine or squirt some back into the bottle until the right amount is in the syringe.

How to give an intramuscular or 'IM' injection

Most medicines are injected into muscle, by intramuscular or IM injection. In an IM injection the medicine goes into the muscle or meat of the animal, in the rump or in the neck. Vaccinations are usually given into the neck muscle. Very thin animals should always be injected into the rump.

WHERE TO INJECT

First, be able to feel the bony points labelled in the picture. Also, think where in the neck the spine is, also shown in the picture. The parts of bones that can be felt are shaded black in the picture.

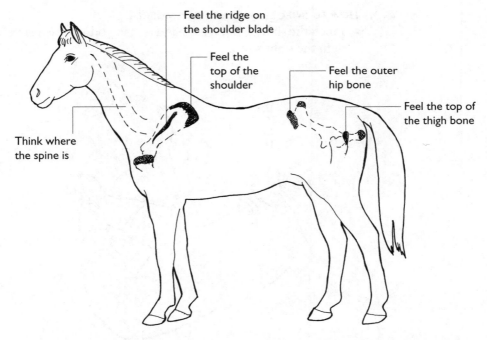

Feel the ridge on the shoulder blade

Feel the top of the shoulder

Feel the outer hip bone

Feel the top of the thigh bone

Think where the spine is

For a neck IM injection, put the needle into the middle of an imaginary triangle bounded by the spine, the shoulder blade and the top of the neck.

For a rump IM injection, aim for the middle of an imaginary square bounded by the point of the hip, the top of the thigh bone, the base of the tail and the back bone.

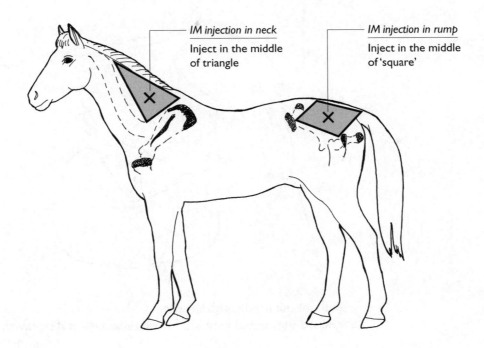

IM injection in neck
Inject in the middle of triangle

IM injection in rump
Inject in the middle of 'square'

HOW TO INJECT INTO THE NECK MUSCLE

- Pinch the skin with the left hand and introduce the needle slowly with the right hand.

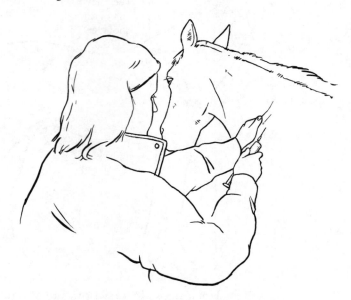

- Try to suck back to make sure the needle is not in a blood vessel and, if you see blood come into the syringe, take the needle out and start again.
- Firmly squeeze the plunger to inject the medicine into the muscle.

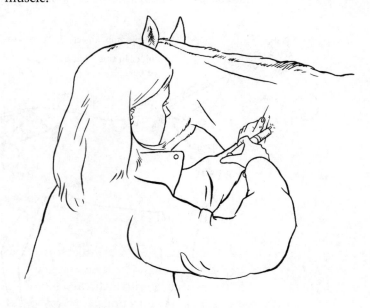

- Pull out the needle, rub the site.
- Reward the animal with kind words and a pat if it behaved.

HOW TO INJECT INTO THE RUMP ('GLUTEAL MUSCLES')

- Choose a clean area of skin (if you have surgical spirit and cotton wool, wipe the injection site with it).
- Remove the needle from the syringe (do not touch the needle itself).
- Hold the needle by the base between finger and thumb with the point away from the palm of your hand.
- Lightly slap the back of your hand against the animal's skin twice.

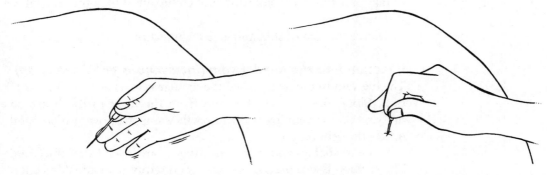

- On the third slap, turn your hand and slap the point of the needle in right to the base of the needle.
- Attach the syringe to the needle.

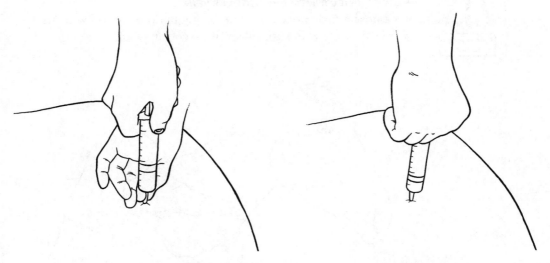

- Continue with the other steps as for injecting into the neck.

Subcutaneous or 'SC' injection

In a subcutaneous injection, medicine is injected just under the skin of the animal. Some medicines, tetanus antitoxin and some vaccines are given as SC injections.

The place for a subcutaneous injection is the skin on the side of the neck.

HOW TO INJECT UNDER THE SKIN

- Choose a clean area of skin (if you have surgical spirit and cotton wool, wipe the injection site with it).
- Pinch a fold of skin.
- Keep the needle attached to the syringe.
- Push the needle into the tent of pinched skin.
- Keep the syringe flat against the animal's body so the needle does not go into the muscle.
- Take care that the needle does not come out of the other side of the skin fold.
- Release the fold of skin and give the injection.

Injection into the jugular vein (intravenous or 'IV' injection)

The big vein in the neck, called the jugular vein, is used for IV injection. Blood flows down this vein from the head to the heart, so pressing on the vein lower down partly dams the flow of blood and makes the vein bigger.

Some medicines and many anaesthetics are given by IV injection. The method is also used for taking blood samples. In an IV injection the needle goes into the animal's blood in the big neck vein. Be sure that the equipment, the animal's skin and your hands are very clean.

Get trained helper!

HOW TO INJECT INTO THE JUGULAR VEIN

- Choose a clean area of skin in the jugular groove and wipe the injection site with surgical spirit on cotton wool.

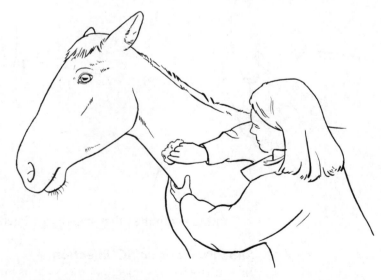

- Have the animal's head held so the neck is straight or turned slightly away from the side on which the injection will be made (to help remove slack folds in the skin).
- Put your thumb in the groove to make the vein stand out.

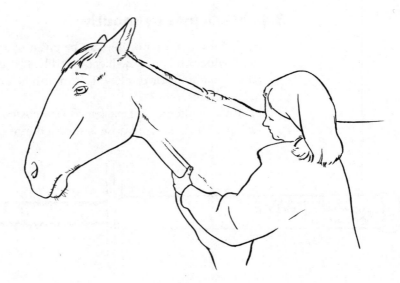

- By tapping the vein it is possible to see or feel a fluid wave that helps locate the vein.
- Direct the needle up the vein, and push it through the skin.
- If you have put the needle in at right angles to the skin, it may pass straight through the vein, so pull it back slightly.
- Pull back the plunger and dark blood will flow into the syringe when the needle is in the vein.

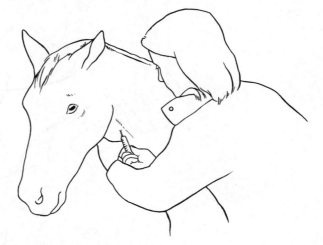

- Stop pressing the vein with your thumb.
- Inject medication slowly.
- Periodically, check that the needle is still in the vein by pulling back on the plunger and looking for blood coming into the syringe.

If taking a blood sample, do not stop pressing with your thumb until you have collected the amount of blood needed.

3.4 Medicines by mouth

Medicines that are powder can be given by mixing with tasty, moist food, which the horse will eat greedily. It is difficult to give a pill or tablet to a horse or donkey. The mouth is long and there is a risk of being bitten.

Some medicines are packaged as a paste in a plastic 'dial-a-dose' syringe. The measured dose is squirted into the back of the mouth.

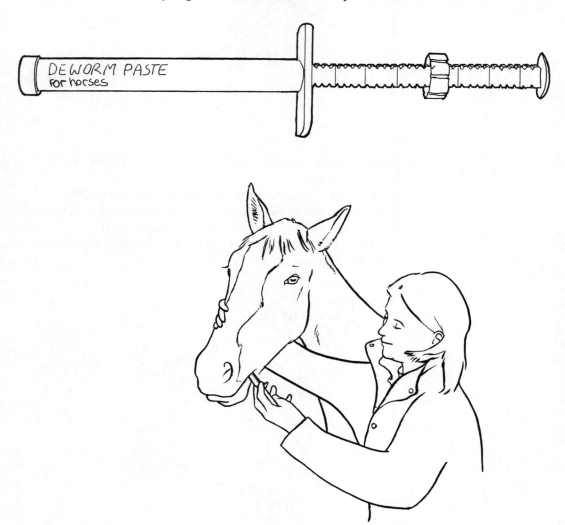

To make a paste syringe cut the end off a normal plastic syringe. Mix the medicine to make a sticky paste.

Be very careful about giving horses and donkeys medicines from a bottle. There is danger of biting the bottle and breaking the glass. Put a piece of plastic or rubber pipe on the neck of the bottle. Also, be careful to allow the horse time to swallow properly.

3.5 How to use a stomach tube

A stomach tube is used to get liquids
into the animal's stomach. The tube is
pushed up the animal's nose. Before
using a stomach tube for the first time,
get training from an experienced
person.

Use a smooth tube with the correct
bore (diameter <2 cm). A funnel can be
attached to the end.

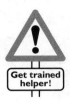

Get trained
helper!

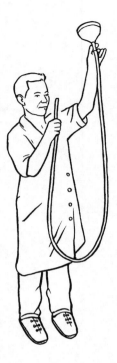

HOW TO PASS A STOMACH TUBE
- Hold the tube beside the horse. Make
  a mark on the tube with a pen to
  show roughly how much of the tube
  needs to go in to reach the stomach.

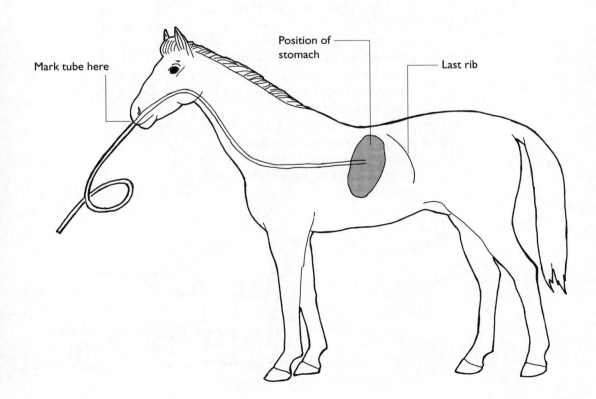

Mark tube here

Position of
stomach

Last rib

- If the tube is stiff, soak it in hot water to soften it.
- Put petroleum jelly on the tube to lubricate it.
- Place tube in the bottom of the nose.

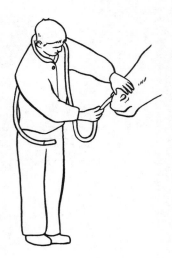

- Keep the horse's neck flexed, but not too much.
- Introduce the tube slowly until you feel the horse swallowing.
- Push on slowly.
- Blow down the tube every 10 cm of tube that goes in to open the path for the tube. Then suck: you should feel resistance provided the tube is going the right way to the stomach. If the stomach tube is going the wrong way, to the lungs, you will suck air back and the animal may cough.

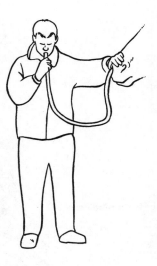

- Watch for the tube in the groove on the left side of the neck, as it passes down towards the stomach. Feel the end of the tube go past your fingers held in the groove on the side of the neck.
- Feel the tube go more easily and smell gas when the tube enters the stomach.
- If you have passed the mark put on the tube before the start, do not push too much more of the tube inside.
- With the tube in place, liquid can be poured into the stomach down a funnel attached to the tube. Hold the funnel high so the liquid runs into the stomach.

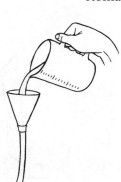

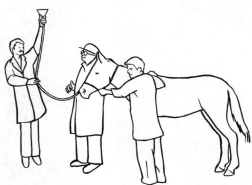

- After giving the medicine, gently pull out the tube.
- If you fold the end of the tube in half as you pull it out, this will stop any liquid left in the tube from running out as the end of the tube comes out past the animal's throat.

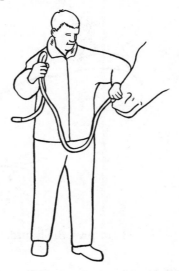

3.6 How to spray medicine on to skin

For treating skin parasites and some other diseases of skin, a small sprayer is useful. The medicine is mixed with water according to the manufacturer's instructions. Take care not to spill the chemical on your own skin. Wear plastic gloves or put your hands in polythene bags before starting.

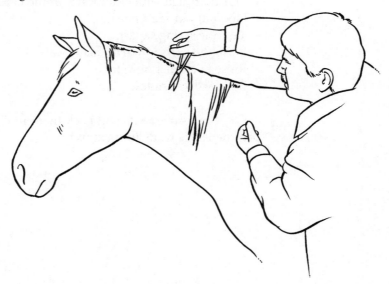

First, clip the hair so that the medicine can reach the affected areas.

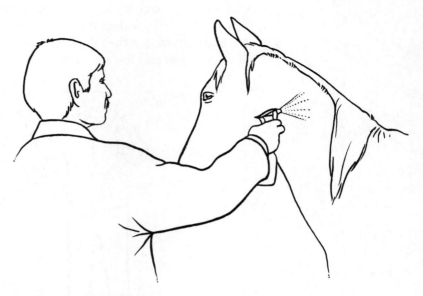

Then spray the liquid.

3.7 How to sterilize equipment

Any instrument that pierces the skin must be very clean before use. Equipment must be boiled in water for 10 minutes to be sure there is no chance of it carrying infection to an animal.

Cleaning syringes and needles:

- Flush through with clean water immediately after using (never let blood dry inside a needle).
- Take the syringe apart.
- Wash the parts in warm, soapy water.
- Rinse in clean, hot water.
- Boil for 10 minutes.

Dry the instruments and pack them in clean paper or in a clean polythene bag ready for next use.

4

Normal feet and legs and shoeing

4.1 Normal feet and legs

Normal feet

The hoof is the horny covering of the foot. The foot means the hoof and everything inside the hoof. The hoof wall is insensitive and nails can be driven through this part without causing pain. Names of parts of the foot, which are used in this book, are labelled on the pictures of the horse's foot.

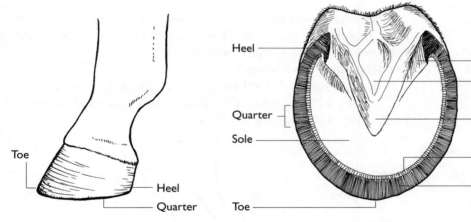

Side view of horse foot

Ground surface of horse foot

A donkey's foot is more upright than a horse's foot and has a different shape. Because of this the sole has a different shape.

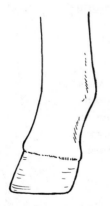

Side view of donkey foot

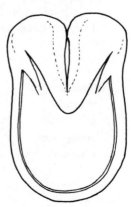

Ground surface of donkey foot

Normal legs

The shape of normal legs is shown in these pictures.

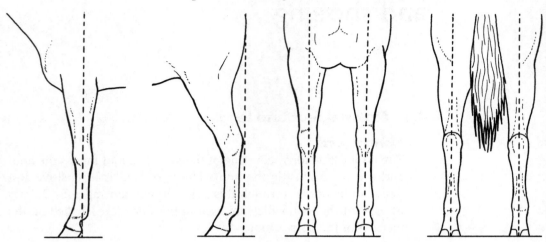

Differences from these 'ideal' leg shapes may be due to wrong bone growth, wrong posture, or injury. Defects of leg shape due to bone growth can sometimes be corrected by trimming the hooves to restore balance in the leg.

It is important to know that the hoof and pastern should be in line, as shown in the picture.(The pastern is the joint just above the hoof, between the foot and the fetlock.)

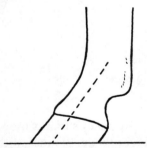

The straight line is lost if the hoof is trimmed too much at the front or back, as shown in these pictures.

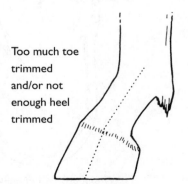

Too much toe
trimmed
and/or not
enough heel
trimmed

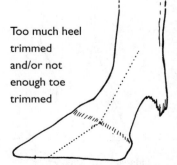

Too much heel
trimmed
and/or not
enough toe
trimmed

Routine hoof care

Animals working without shoes should have their feet checked every four weeks or sooner.

The hoof tends to split at the edges and spread at the ground, especially at the quarters. Rasping the edge of the hoof can reduce this.

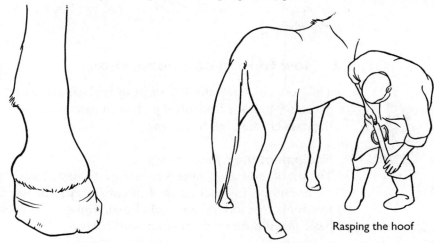

Hoof with splaying edge

Rasping the hoof

Be sure that an animal without shoes is not becoming foot-sore because the wall is wearing too fast on the road. If so, shoes should be put on.

Feet should have dirt picked out of the sole and frog with a hoof pick every morning and evening.

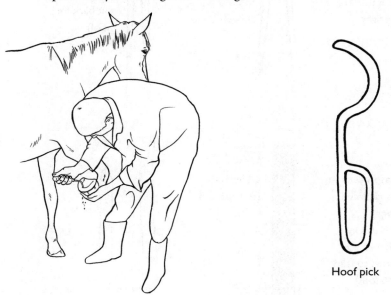

Hoof pick

In hot, dry seasons, a hoof may become too dry and then get hard and crack. Moisture can be put back into a hoof by washing daily with water. Use a very soft brush in order that the outer layer of the hoof is not damaged. Alternatively stand the animal in a shallow pool or stream for a few minutes each day until the hooves become softer and less brittle.

Sometimes oils are painted on hooves. Oils can be useful. Hoof oil forms a barrier that keeps moisture in, but in the same way the oil keeps water out. Therefore, do not use hoof oil on dry, brittle hooves.

4.2 How to replace a horse shoe

Get trained helper!

This section shows the key steps in replacing a horse's shoe. It is necessary to learn from an experienced person and to practise with their supervision when learning.

Equipment used for shoeing

The list of tools given here is typical of the basic tools used by farriers in Europe. In other parts of the world, farriers may use alternative tools to some of the tools listed. However, the principles of basic shoeing are valid whatever tools are used.

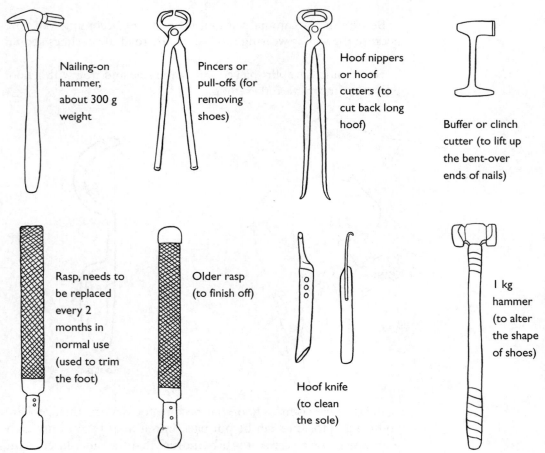

Nailing-on hammer, about 300 g weight

Pincers or pull-offs (for removing shoes)

Hoof nippers or hoof cutters (to cut back long hoof)

Buffer or clinch cutter (to lift up the bent-over ends of nails)

Rasp, needs to be replaced every 2 months in normal use (used to trim the foot)

Older rasp (to finish off)

Hoof knife (to clean the sole)

1 kg hammer (to alter the shape of shoes)

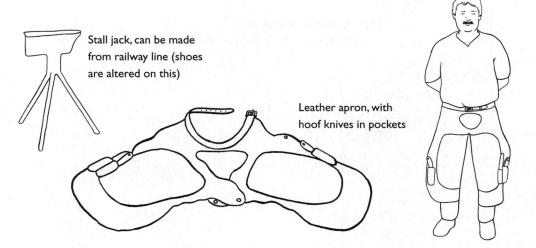

Stall jack, can be made from railway line (shoes are altered on this)

Leather apron, with hoof knives in pockets

For making horseshoes, extra tools and equipment are needed. These are described in specialist books about horseshoeing.

How to hold the foot
Pick up the horse's foot.
Step over the foot, and grip the leg between your thighs.

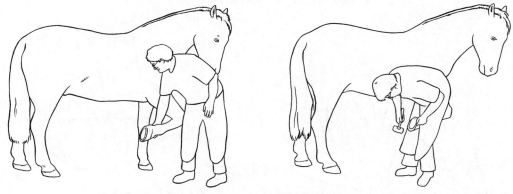

When shoeing a donkey, the donkey's leg is held lower than a horse's leg, because a donkey is smaller than a horse. If the donkey's leg were held between the thighs, as a horse's foot would be, the donkey's leg would be twisted.

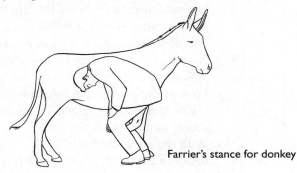

Farrier's stance for donkey

How to remove a shoe
- Straighten or break the turned-over part of all the nails.

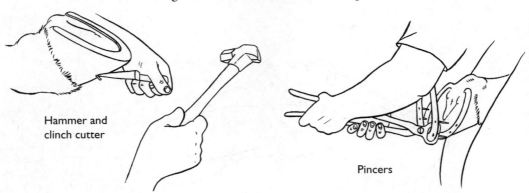

Hammer and clinch cutter

Pincers

- Use the pincers to lever off the shoe, starting at the inside heel. Push the handles of the pincers down and in towards the toe of the foot. Work first down one side, then down the other side. To help get leverage it is important to support the foot at the same time.

How to trim the hoof
- Remove loose flakes of sole with the knife.

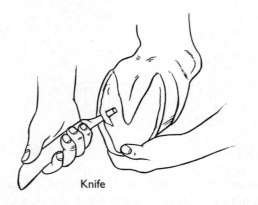

Knife

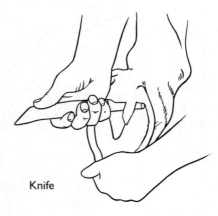

Knife

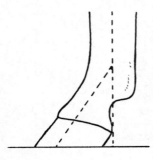

- Trim the edges of the frog with the knife.
- When trimming the hoof, the aim is to make the shape like that of the normal foot, described above. After shoeing, the pastern and hoof should be at the same angle. If the heel is not trimmed enough, the hoof becomes too upright. This can result in lameness.
- Look at the hoof and decide how much to trim. After trimming, the hoof should be balanced on each side and the hoof walls should not be below the level of the wide part of the frog.
- With the knife, cut back the sole around the white line to the depth of the hoof wall that is to be removed.

- Starting at one heel, cut round the hoof wall with hoof nippers to shorten the foot.

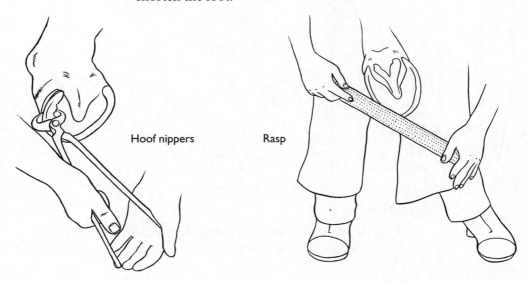

Hoof nippers   Rasp

- Rasp the sole flat and even.
- Check that the hoof and the pastern are in a straight line.

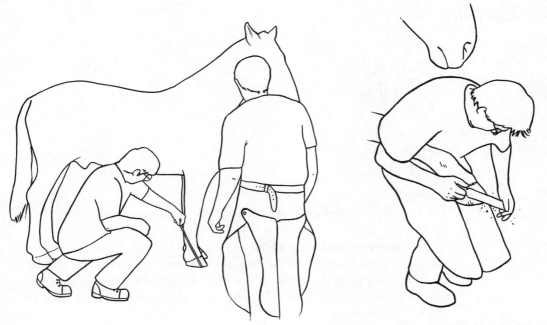

Rasp outside of hoof wall

- Alter shape of foot if necessary.
- Rasp the outside edge so the wall has even thickness at the ground. Do not rasp the shiny outside of the wall high up the hoof.

How to make the new shoe the correct size

- Measure across the foot in three places and select the correct size of shoe.

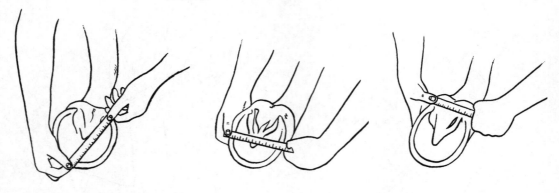

- If necessary, make the shoe wider to fit the foot, using the hammer and stall jack.

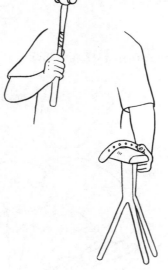
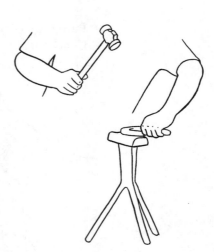

- Flatten the shoe, again using the hammer and stall jack.

How to nail on a shoe

- When nailing on the shoe, imagine, or draw, a line one quarter to one third up the hoof. The nails should come out at this line.
- Position the point of the nail in the horn of the wall outside the white line.
- If using proper horseshoe nails, face the nail bevel to the frog.

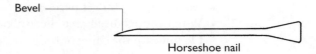

Bevel

Horseshoe nail

- Hold the shoe hard and hammer the nail, aiming for the imaginary or drawn line.

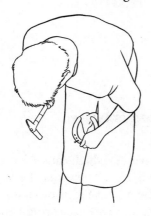 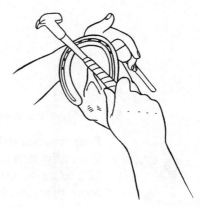

- Hammer nails against pincers to tighten them.
- Clip the ends of the nails with the pincers so that 3 mm of nail sticks out from the hoof wall.

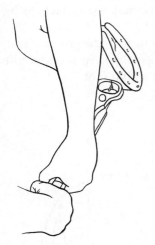 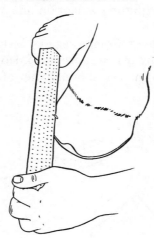 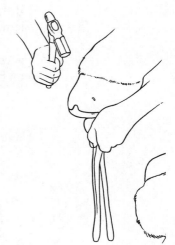

- Using the rasp, make a groove under the end of the nail that sticks out.
- Hammer the nail against the pincers to turn the nail end over into the groove.

To remove a nail, for example because it has been driven in the wrong place.

- Straighten the end of the nail if it is bent over.
- Hammer on the shoe either side of the head of the nail.
- Hold the closed pincers against the point of the nail and push the nail.
- When enough of the nail head is above the hoof, pull it out with the pincers.

5 Lameness

5.1 How to decide which leg is lame

Get trained helper!

Professional advice

It is difficult to decide where the pain is which causes lameness. It is best to get an experienced vet to decide. There may be lameness in more than one leg. There may be an earlier, root cause that over time has resulted in other lameness. Always get professional advice when possible.

First, look at the standing, resting animal

If it is not putting weight on one of its legs, that one is likely to be lame.

The foot of the lame leg may be held pointing to the ground. This is especially true of a front leg. Horses normally keep their weight on both front feet, although they often rest a hind foot.

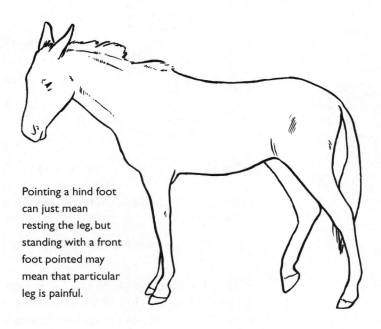

Pointing a hind foot can just mean resting the leg, but standing with a front foot pointed may mean that particular leg is painful.

After a horse has been lame on one of its fore legs for a long time, the leg may straighten.

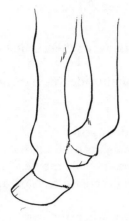

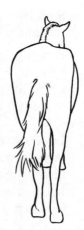

A horse that has been lame for a long time may have less muscle on the lame side. From behind the horse, look for differences in the amount of muscle on the quarters. Look for a difference in the amount of muscle over the shoulders on each side.

Look for new swellings, especially around joints.

Look for swellings over tendons, particularly at the back of the cannon of the front leg, as shown in the next picture.

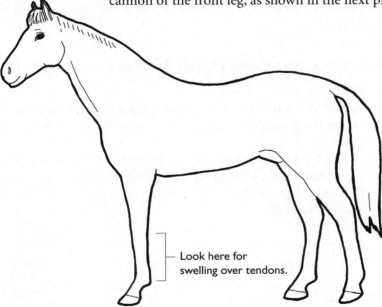

Look here for swelling over tendons.

Pick the feet up

Pick up all four feet in turn and clean the dirt out of the soles. Look for injury, discharges, stones, bruising and nails.

Look at the animal trotting away from you

Get someone to *trot* the animal away from you for 20 metres on level, hard ground. Watch each hip to see if it goes up or down when the hind foot hits the ground.

- Both hips stay almost level in a horse when there is no hind leg lameness.
- The hip goes up and down more on the side where there is pain in that hind leg.

Look at the animal trotting towards you

When it trots, look for the horse moving its head up as its front foot hits the ground. A normal horse does not lift the head much. If a horse moves its head up, it is usually because it feels pain in a front leg when it takes weight.

The animal will nod its head down when the front foot on the good side hits the ground. The animal tries to take more weight on the good side. Remember, *when the lame animal trots, it nods on the good leg.* Its head nods down when the front leg hits the ground on the side opposite to the lame leg.

Look at the trotting animal from the side too. An animal lame in both hind legs tends to take short steps, and may drag the toes of its feet along the ground (look for wear on the toes).Usually lifting the head is a sign of front leg lameness, but it can indicate severe pain in a hind leg.

5.2   Checking more closely for the source of lameness

Feet

Always check the feet very carefully. Most lameness is in the feet. A farrier (blacksmith) is often experienced at finding problem areas in a foot.

Feel for heat. Always compare the suspected problem side with the opposite one. If one foot feels much hotter, this suggests infection or broken foot bones. If there is heat in the feet on both sides, it suggests laminitis.

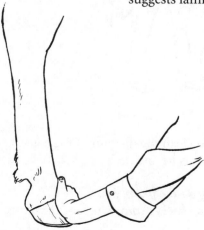
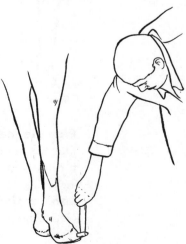

Pick up the foot and look underneath. Press as hard as you can with your thumbs and see if the animal shows pain by trying to pull its foot away. If you are not sure if there is pain, use a hammer or hoof tester tool. See the section *Nail through the sole and infection in the foot.*

The coronary band area

Feel the area just above the wall of the hoof for pain and swelling. Swelling at the front or back of this area may suggest tendon damage. Swelling at the back may be caused by infection coming up from the foot. Feel the cartilages (see the sections *Quittor* and *Ring bone*).

Shins

Feel for pain by rubbing the front of the shins firmly with a clenched fist. Pain suggests sore shins. You may notice 'splints' which are bony swellings on the shin bones. See the sections *Sore shins* and *Splints.*

Tendons

Injuries to the tendons cause heat and pain and swelling. Carefully feel the area behind the cannon (shin) bone. The place to check is shown in the drawing in the previous section.

Joints

Feel for heat in all the joints from the fetlock joint up to the shoulder or hip. The names of joints used in this book are shown in the picture.

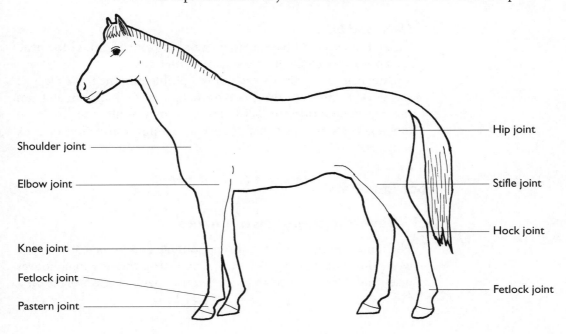

Shoulder joint

Elbow joint

Knee joint

Fetlock joint

Pastern joint

Hip joint

Stifle joint

Hock joint

Fetlock joint

Fetlocks

Swellings behind the fetlock joints without heat or pain are common. They are sometimes called 'windgalls' and are not normally serious in older animals. Pain and heat can sometimes suggest a serious problem, such as damage to ligaments or to the pair of small bones behind the joint.

Knees

Heat and swelling in the knee follows injury to the (carpal) bones in the knee or the ligaments which connect them. Swelling can also occur around tendons (the cords which connect muscles to bones) where they cross the front or back of the knee. Hard swellings on the front suggest old arthritis.

Elbows

Swelling behind the elbow sometimes occurs (see the section *Capped elbow*).

Hocks

Look for soft swelling at the front and inside of the joint (see the section *Bog spavin*). Hard, bony enlargement may be felt at the inside of the joint (see the section *Bone spavin*).

Stifle

The connections between bones (called ligaments) of this joint are sometimes injured, causing pain in the joint and lameness. The leg may become stiff and straight if the joint gets 'locked'.

Neck and back

Check the neck and back as well. Stand in front and hold the head up. Look for swelling on one side of the neck.

Lameness is not always caused by a problem in the feet or legs. If the neck is injured, the pain from this stops the animal from moving its neck freely. Injury to the spine may result in the back not looking as straight as usual because of strong contraction of back muscles on one side.

Foot lameness

5.3 Severely overgrown hooves

The hoof continues to grow throughout life and in the natural state wears down as it grows. Sometimes animals grow very long hooves when they are rested or injured, because they put less weight on a foot.

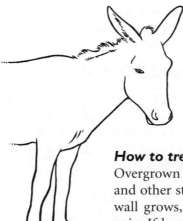

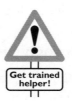

Get trained
helper!

How to treat overgrown hooves

Overgrown hooves can be trimmed quite boldly because the bones and other structures inside the hoof do not grow down as the hoof wall grows, and because overgrown hoof wall is not sensitive to pain. If hooves are very overgrown, it is best to trim back the hoof to the normal shape in more than one session, allowing two weeks between each session.

The aim is to restore the hoof to its normal shape and angle to the ground. See the section *Normal feet and legs* for the normal angle of the hoof to the ground. The section *How to replace a horseshoe* also explains how to trim a hoof.

- Using a sharp knife cut the sole back. Press with your thumbs to make sure that the sole is firm. Stop cutting the sole as soon as you feel a little tiny bit of movement of the sole under thumb pressure. Immediately stop cutting deeper if you see a pinkish colour or blood.

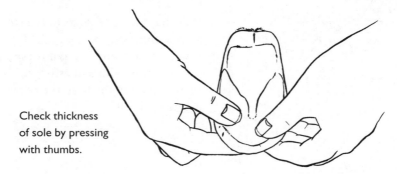

Check thickness of sole by pressing with thumbs.

- After cutting the sole, use hoof cutters to remove the overgrown wall. Remember the hoof wall bears the weight, not the sole. Therefore, the hoof wall is trimmed so that it remains longer than the sole.
- When cutting the wall, it is necessary to keep comparing both sides to make sure that they are balanced and symmetric.
- Use a rasp to tidy up, but be very careful not to take off too much hoof wall with the rasp.
- Use a sharp knife to trim the frog. After trimming, it should have its normal shape and should just contact the ground.

- After trimming, make sure the animal stands in a place with deep, clean bedding such as straw for at least a week.

5.4   Nail through the sole and infection in the foot

Nails and other sharp objects sometimes get trodden on and penetrate the sole. A horseshoe nail in the wrong place can also cause infection. If infection develops, the horse is in great pain. If infection becomes established in the joints inside the foot or the tendons, it may never be cured in some cases.

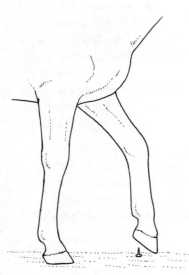

What infection in the foot looks like
- The animal will not be willing to put the foot on the ground.
- It may stand with the affected foot pointed down to the ground, not resting weight on it.
- The foot feels hot.
- Pain usually increases after a few days when infection gets worse.

How to decide if there is something painful in the foot and find the painful place
- Pick up the foot and look for a 'foreign body'. It is often possible to see a nail or the end of a piece of metal. If you do not see anything, it may have gone deeper into the foot.
- Press hard over all parts of the sole, and see if the animal flinches.
- If you are not sure of a pain response, tap round the sole and wall with a hammer or the handle of a knife. If there is pain in the foot, the horse will immediately lift it when it is hit.

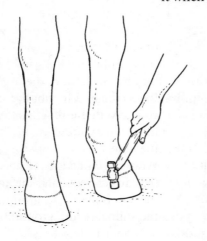

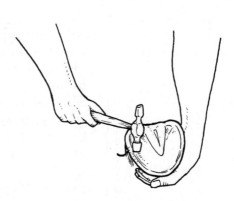

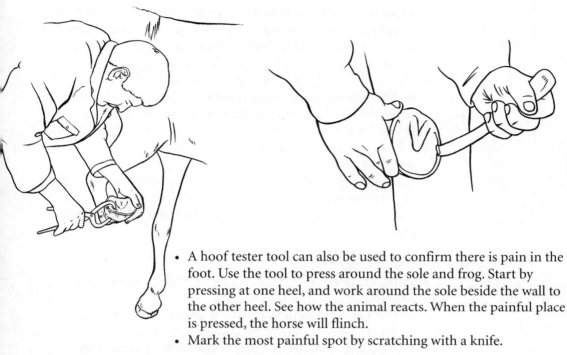

- A hoof tester tool can also be used to confirm there is pain in the foot. Use the tool to press around the sole and frog. Start by pressing at one heel, and work around the sole beside the wall to the other heel. See how the animal reacts. When the painful place is pressed, the horse will flinch.
- Mark the most painful spot by scratching with a knife.

How to treat infection in the foot

TETANUS INJECTION
Check if the animal is vaccinated against tetanus. If not, inject with tetanus antitoxin.

TREAT THE FOOT

Get trained helper!

- Pull out the nail or other object if you can see it.
- With a sharp knife, open up the track where the object entered. Farriers or blacksmiths are usually the best people to get to do this. If you could not see the end of a nail, the track is likely to be in the place where there was greatest pain.

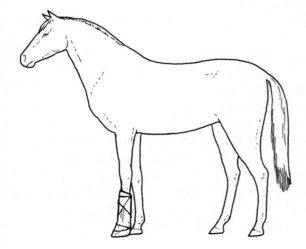

  - It is important to cut out enough of the sole to let all the infection out, or else the infection will come back. If in doubt, make the hole a bit bigger.
  - Use syringes full of boiled and cooled water to flush out the infection by squirting the fluid into the hole.
  - Wrap the foot with a clean sack so that dirt cannot enter the hole when the foot is put to the ground. Keep the animal on dry ground.

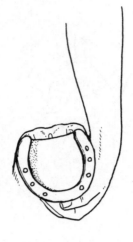

- Remove the sack two or three times each day and soak the foot in a bucket of warm, salty water (as hot as you can comfortably bear your own hands in) for about 10 minutes. Dry the foot and replace the sack. Do this for a week.
- If there is no more pus, no pain, and the horse walks on the foot without lameness, pack cotton wool (unspun cotton) with 'Stockholm tar' or with antiseptic ointment into the hole.
- Do not let the horse stand on dirty, wet ground.
- Leather across the sole helps protect it. The leather is put over the sole when nailing on a shoe.
- After another ten days, cut the piece of leather around the inside of the shoe.
- Keep the horse on dry ground for the next few days and then gradually bring it back to normal work.

ANTIBIOTIC INJECTIONS
- When the infection is drained fully, antibiotics are not necessary or helpful.
- Only if the horse has a fever the day after the infection is cut out of the foot, give antibiotic injections for three days.
- Infections deep in the foot may temporarily improve with antibiotics but, if the joints or tendons in the foot are affected, these infections may never improve. Some animals remain extremely lame and have to be euthanased because they cannot be cured.

5.5   Laminitis

Laminitis is inflammation under the horny wall of the hoof. An animal with acute laminitis is extremely lame and uncomfortable.

What causes laminitis
- Some allergies or digestive problems,
- eating a lot of lush grass – especially small, fat ponies taking too little exercise,
- eating a lot of grain such as wheat,
- retained afterbirth (see the section *Retained placenta* in the chapter *Birth and care of foals*),
- a lot of work on hard ground.

What acute (i.e. sudden onset) laminitis looks like
- The affected feet feel hotter around the coronary band.
- The animal is very lame, and reluctant to put weight on affected feet. This may make it stand in an unusual way, appearing to lean back on its heels.
- The sole may bulge due to pressure in the foot.

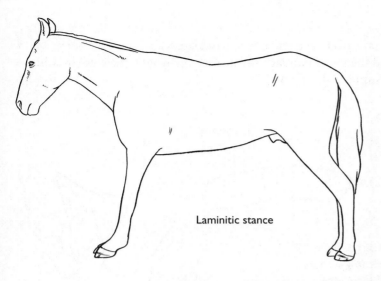

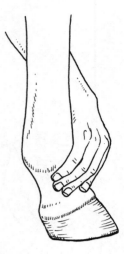

Laminitic stance

- The pulse can be felt more strongly than normal in blood vessels above the foot. See the section on *Temperature, heart rate and breathing*.

How to treat sudden onset laminitis

STOP ANY DIETARY CAUSE

If diet is the cause, stop the animal eating grain or similar. Give a laxative, for example, 500 ml of liquid paraffin, so that the bad food passes through the horse faster. See the section *About poisons and general treatment* for medicines to make food pass through more quickly.

MAKE THE FEET MORE COMFORTABLE

- Provide a deep, soft bed.
- Put sand on the stable floor.
- Let the horse stand in cool water or mud, for example, in a stream, three or four times a day.
- Do not remove horse shoes because the sole may be painful. (Only remove shoes if nails placed too deeply appear to be causing the problem.)

GIVE SUPPORT TO THE FROG

The aim of a frog support is to transfer more weight from the hoof walls to the frog. To make it you need a roll of strong, sticky tape and a rolled bandage 8 or 10 cm wide.

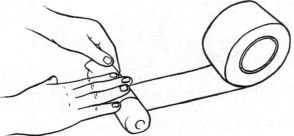

- Roll sticky tape around the bandage.

- Put tape over each end of the bandage.
- Hold the taped bandage roll against the frog to measure how big the support should be.

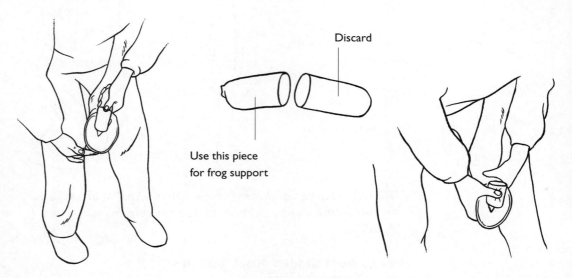

Discard

Use this piece
for frog support

- Cut the support to the required length with a very sharp knife, for example, a scalpel blade.
- Put strips of tape over the cut end and again wind tape around it.
- Hold it on the frog.
- Use strips of tape to fix it to the sole and walls of the hoof.
- Finish off with sticky tape around the walls of the hoof. Do not stick tape on to hair, only on to the hoof wall.
- Keep the frog support in place for two weeks.

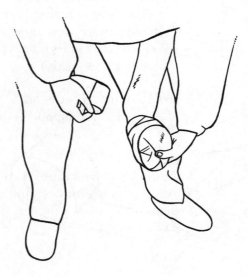

DRUGS TO REDUCE PAIN AND INFLAMMATION
- Phenylbutazone or other NSAID type drugs.
- Do not give corticosteroid drugs.

If the tip of the bone that is normally inside the hoof can be seen poking through the sole of the foot, the foot will not recover. Euthanasia is recommended.

How to treat laminitis later, after the foot has changed shape
FOOT TRIMMING

Get trained helper!

After some time, laminitis changes the shape of the foot. The wall becomes longer at the heel. Trimming is needed to correct this.

- Check the sole for infection. Abscesses are often found near the tip of the frog. Find the infected place and treat by cutting the sole as described in the section, *Nail through the sole and infection in the foot.*
- Trim the toe back to the white zone. The white line (see the section *Normal feet and legs*) becomes wider because of laminitis. At the toe the white line may be 2 cm wide. The lower part of the wall at the toe is rasped off down to the white line.
- Trim the heel to make it near the length it would be on a normal foot.

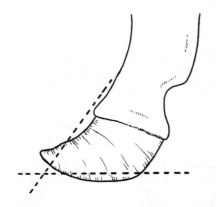
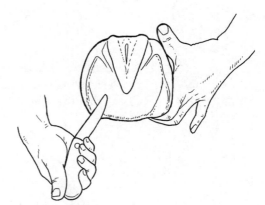

After the toe has been rasped away, a blacksmith may fit a special shoe, for example, a shoe made with a clip at each quarter instead of one clip at the toe.

DIET

If eating lush grass caused laminitis, the animal should be kept away from the grass, housed, and given a little hay each day. When it seems better, allow a maximum of one hour to graze each day for at least a month.

5.6 Bruised sole and 'corns'

When the sole is bruised there is bleeding beneath the surface. Soreness and pressure in the foot causes pain and lameness.

A corn is a bruise on the sole between wall and bars in the position shown in the picture. Horses usually get corns on the front feet when wearing shoes.

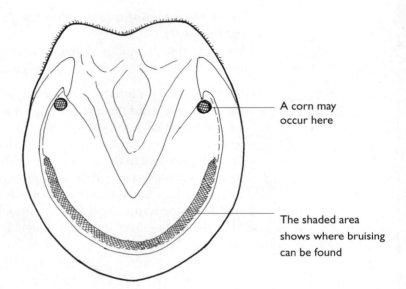

A corn may occur here

The shaded area shows where bruising can be found

Causes of bruises on the sole

- Leaving shoes on too long. The wall of the hoof may grow long so that the sole of the foot presses on the back parts of the shoe,

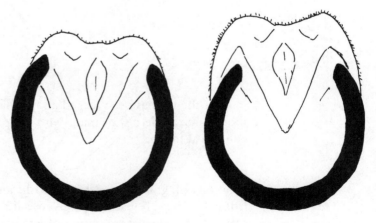

(a) A well fitted shoe.

(b) This shoe has been left on too long. The hoof wall has grown. Now part of the sole presses on the heels of the shoe and corns can result.

- bad shoeing,
- stone under the shoe,
- work on hard roads,
- jumping on to stones or hard objects.

What bruised sole looks like
- Lameness.
- Bruising which at first shows as bleeding under the sole.
- Later the bruised area looks yellow and the sole is flaky.
- The affected area is just inside the walls (nails are more often beside the frog).

How to prevent bruised soles
- Proper, regular shoeing. Do not leave shoes on too long.
- Check feet daily and pick out debris and stones.

How to treat mild cases of bruised sole
- Remove the shoe.
- Rest the horse and give soft bedding.
- If the animal has to keep working place a leather pad across the sole (see the section *Nail through the sole and infection in the foot*).

How to treat severe cases of bruised sole with infection
This is a job for the farrier or blacksmith.

Get trained helper!

- With a knife, pare off the surface layers of the sole, and look for signs of bruising and infection.

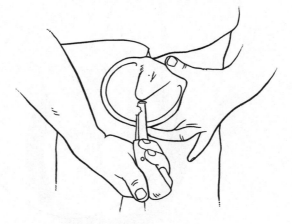

- Cut out the bruised area.
- If there is infection, cut away to allow drainage, as for nail in the foot, and stand the foot in hot, salty water twice daily for three days. If the animal has a fever, give antibiotic injections for three days.

- Inject tetanus antitoxin.
- A set-heeled shoe can be fitted to prevent weight being carried on the area with the corn.

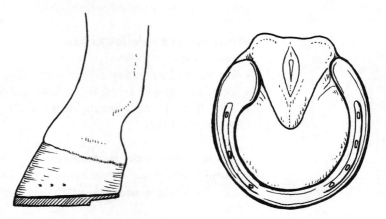

5.7 Hoof cracks

Cracks are common when horses without shoes do not have their feet trimmed. The end of the hoof wall grows out and splits.

When you see a crack in a hoof, first look at the sole. If the crack does not cross the whole wall, it is not usually important. Such cracks are sometimes called weather cracks.

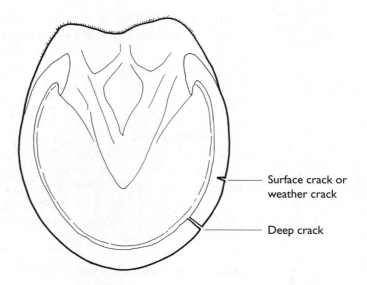

Surface crack or weather crack

Deep crack

When you look at the sole and see a deep crack that goes across all of the hoof wall, it is a true crack. This kind of crack is known as a grass crack or a sand crack depending whether the crack starts at the bottom or the top of the hoof.

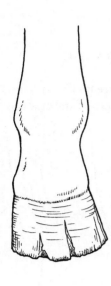

A.   Grass cracks

Cracks often occur after horses are turned out to graze for some time, so they are called 'grass cracks'. A grass crack does not go all the way up to the top of the hoof.

What a grass crack looks like
- Cracks rising up from the sole.
- Usually not lame, unless the crack is big and opens when the animal walks.

How to prevent grass cracks
Keep feet properly trimmed.

How to treat grass cracks
When shoes are put on again, the crack usually grows out and disappears. If the grass crack is severe these treatments help.

- If the hoof is dry and brittle, use a cloth or brush to paint water on the outside of the hoof each day. Alternatively, stand the horse in water, for example, in a stream. Some of the water is absorbed into the hoof.
- A skilled blacksmith can make a shoe with clips each side of the crack.
- Severe grass cracks can be fixed with nails across the crack (see the section *How to treat a deep sand crack*).
- Make the top of the crack wide.
  - with a heated metal rod, burn a hole into the hoof wall at the top of the crack. The hole should be about 1 cm diameter and 0.5 cm deep.
  - or, use a rasp to make a groove at an angle on each side of the crack.

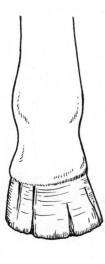

B.   Sand cracks

A crack that starts at the top of the hoof is sometimes called a 'sand crack'. It is usually caused by an injury to the coronary band, from where the hoof grows.

The sides of a sand crack never grow back together. The crack disappears only if new horn starts to grow down from the top of the hoof without splitting.

What sand cracks look like
- A crack starting from the top of the hoof.
- Pain and lameness if it is a deep crack extending right through the hoof wall.
- Blood or pus may exude from deep sand cracks.

How to prevent sand cracks
Avoid injury to the top of the hoof.

How to treat a sand crack that does not go through all layers of the hoof
Cut grooves into the hoof each side of the crack (see pictures). These grooves help reduce the movement between the sides of the crack.

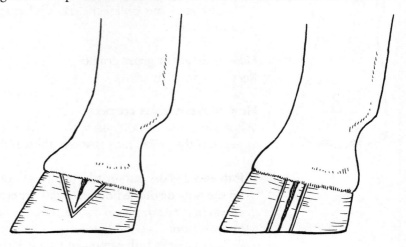

How to treat a deep sand crack
Put nails across the crack to stop the crack's sides from moving.

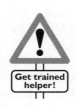

Get trained helper!

- With a hot metal rod, burn dents in the hoof either side of the crack.
- Drive a small horseshoe nail across the crack, taking great care not to go too deep, and tap the head of the nail as far as it will go.
- Turn the end of the nail over and cut off excess length.
- Repeat so there are two or three nails across the crack.

Do not remove these nails. Leave them in until they eventually grow out as the horn of the hoof grows down.

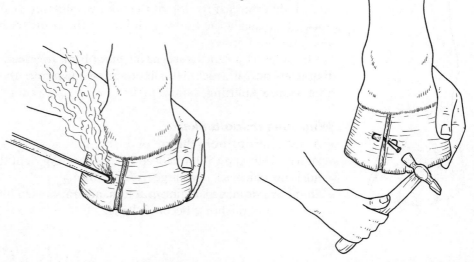

5.8 'Seedy toe'

A seedy toe occurs when the wall separates from the sole at the toe. Small stones and dirt fill the space and in time are pushed up more deeply under the wall of the hoof. Seedy toe sometimes follows laminitis or bruising.

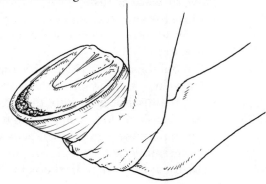

What seedy toe looks like
- There is no lameness in mild cases, but lameness occurs if it is infected.
- Tapping with a hammer over the affected hoof gives a hollow sound.
- When the hoof is picked up, dirt and grit are found just inside the wall.

How to prevent seedy toe
- Trim the wall of overgrown hooves.
- Use a hoof pick regularly to pick stones and dirt out of feet.

How to treat seedy toe
- Remove all dirt with a hoof pick and trim the foot.
- Pack the cavity with cotton wool and Stockholm tar.
- Alternatively, pack with cotton wool and antiseptic ointment.
- Put a new shoe on, over the impregnated cotton.

5.9 Thrush

Thrush is a disease of the frog. This part of the sole decays and has a characteristic, bad smell. Thrush occurs when animals are not looked after properly. Keeping a horse in dirty, wet places causes thrush.

What thrush looks like
- Moist, rotting frog,
- nasty smell,
- sometimes a black discharge from the frog,
- there is no lameness at first, but if no action is taken infection spreads and the horse becomes lame.

How to prevent thrush
- Keep the stable dry and clean.
- Do not make horses stand for long periods on wet ground.
- Pick the feet out regularly.

How to treat thrush
- Move the animal so it does not stand in a wet place. A lot of dry, clean straw on the floor of the stable will help keep the sole of the foot dry.
- Cut out the infected tissue with a sharp knife.
- Each day, scrub the sole with warm, salty water.
- Apply antiseptic daily until the infection has disappeared. Use a paintbrush or cloth to apply it to the affected feet.
- Antiseptics that can be used include copper sulphate solution, a dilute solution of formalin, or potassium permanganate solution. See list at the back of the book for how to dilute and use these antiseptics.

5.10 Canker

Canker is caused in the same way as thrush: by keeping animals on dirty, wet ground . It tends to affect the sole as well as the frog, and the infection tends to track more deeply and can affect the whole of the foot. Treatment may take a long time and is not always successful.

What canker looks like
- A thin, decayed scab-like layer over the sole.
- Under this is a soft, oily, cheesy layer that usually has a bad smell.

How to prevent canker
Prevent canker in the same ways as thrush.

Call vet!

How to treat canker
Canker is difficult to treat. If possible, seek help from a veterinarian because an anaesthetic may be necessary.

- Remove all the diseased tissue with a knife. Some tracks may extend deep into the foot. All diseased sole should be cut out. If the sole bleeds, it may be necessary to bandage the hoof.
- Keep the horse on soft, clean, dry bedding until healthy new horn has grown on the sole of the foot. This may take several months.
- Use antibiotic ointment on the infected sole, binding soaked cotton wool in place with elastic bandage. Change the dressing each day. Instead of ointment, metronidazole solution for injection (Torgyl), or oxytetracycline for injection (Terramycin) can be used to soak the cotton wool.

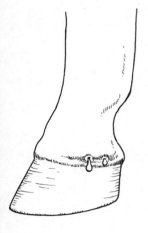

- A course of injections with metronidazole may help recovery. In horses, this drug is given slowly by intravenous injection, once a day for five days.

5.11 Quittor

Quittor is infection deep inside the foot. The infection is in the flexible cartilage plates that can be felt beneath the skin just above the coronary band on each side of the foot. Sometimes the infection discharges pus. See the section *Side bone* for where to feel the cartilage plates.

What quittor looks like
- The horse is very lame.
- Pus discharges just above the coronary band.

How to prevent quittor
It is difficult to prevent. Effective treatment of infection in the sole of the foot may prevent some cases of quittor.

Call vet!

How to treat quittor
Successful treatment usually requires surgery by a veterinarian, who will cut out infected cartilage under general anaesthetic, and use antibiotics against the infection.

5.12 Loss of whole hoof wall

Sometimes an accident can result in the whole hoof wall coming off. The animal is in great pain, the sensitive parts of the hoof are unprotected, and it bleeds a lot.

It would take months for the whole hoof wall to grow again. Before that happens, there is great pain and a strong possibility of infection. The hoof is unlikely to grow properly. Euthanasia is the most appropriate action if the whole hoof wall comes off.

5.13 'Side bone' and 'ring bone'

The area shown in black feels springy in a normal foot, but solid in an animal with side bone.

Side bone and ring bone are caused by the foot repeatedly hitting a hard surface like a road.

What side bone looks like
In side bone, the new bone in the cartilage can be felt just above the horny part of the hoof. In this place, normally the top of the cartilage plate feels a little bit springy. When bone has formed there, it feels solid. Lameness is not common, but does occur if a lot of bone has formed.

What ring bone looks like

In ring bone, new bone forms in the pastern area, sometimes higher (around 'pastern joint') and sometimes lower (around 'coffin joint'). It usually occurs in the front legs. The lower place where bone can develop more often affects the nearby joint and so more often causes lameness.

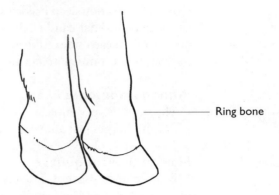

Ring bone

How to treat side bone and ring bone

There is no cure for either side bone or ring bone. To keep an animal with side bone or ring bone as sound as possible:
- Keep the feet trimmed to a proper, balanced shape.
- If there is lameness, relieve pain with anti-inflammatory drugs, for example, phenylbutazone.

How to prevent side bone and ring bone

If you have working animals that suffer from ring bone or side bone (or bony spavin, splints or sore shins), it may be a sign that they have done too much work on hard roads. By making your next animals work less on hard roads, they will remain sound and work longer for you.

5.14 Navicular disease

Navicular disease is a name for changes to a small bone, called the navicular bone, inside the hoof. One or both front legs are affected. Treatment does not eliminate it but controls the lameness caused by it. Experts believe that navicular disease is often part of joint disease affecting other joints as well.

How to recognize navicular disease

- Lameness develops slowly over weeks or months.
- There is a characteristic stiff, quick gait. The horse appears to potter rather than move normally. Lameness may be worse when the animal goes downhill.
- Affected feet may have a more boxy shape and small frog. There is normally pain in the back part of the frog.

- (An experienced veterinarian would take X-rays and do nerve blocks to confirm it is navicular disease.)

How to treat navicular disease
- Make sure that the feet are trimmed properly by the blacksmith, so, for example, the animal does not have long toes. Make sure that the feet and pastern joints are at a normal angle. See the section *Normal feet and legs* for the normal angle of the hoof to the ground.
- Give phenylbutazone, using the smallest dose that causes improvement.

Joint lameness

5.15 Joints swollen for a long time, arthritis

Working horses and donkeys often get swollen joints. Work causes wear to joints. When a joint is worn, it becomes painful. Fluid develops around it causing swelling, which stays even when the animal is rested. This is arthritis. Arthritis cannot normally be cured. Prevention is, therefore, very important.

Following the early swelling, bone slowly builds up around the joint. This can develop slowly for years. Eventually, the joint becomes stuck together with new bone and then it cannot bend any more.

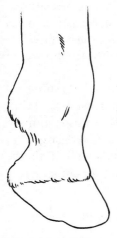

Fetlock joint swollen because of arthritis

How to prevent joint disease
- Think how arthritis in any of your animals may have been caused by the animal's work. Consider how to change or reduce the work done by other animals to prevent joint disease affecting them too. Then they should work longer without getting arthritis.
- Do not make young horses or donkeys work. Wait until they are three years old.
- A wise owner takes action to prevent arthritis. The animal then works better and longer, thus the owner can save money.

5.16 Treatment of swollen joints

The treatment of swollen joints depends on how badly lame the animal is.

How to treat swollen joints if the animal is not lame
- Rest if possible.
- Apply cold compresses. Put ice cubes in a polythene bag and hold it on the swelling, or hold a cloth soaked in cold water on the swollen joint.
- Do not treat with drugs.

- Do not burn the skin with hot irons and do not rub with burning chemicals.

How to treat swollen joints if the animal is moderately lame
- Rest the animal.
- Apply cold compresses.
- Treat with anti-inflammatory drugs, for example, phenylbutazone or ibuprofen.

How to treat a swollen joint if the animal is extremely lame and will not put its foot to the ground
If extremely lame, the animal usually has infection in the joint or a broken bone. The joint feels hot.

- Rest the animal.
- If the body temperature is higher than the normal temperature, give antibiotic injections for at least five days. Start treatment as quickly as you can because infection can damage the surfaces inside the joint in one or two days. Penicillin with streptomycin is recommended.
- Get veterinary help to flush the joint if it is infected. Washing infection from joints is a job for experienced practitioners. Joints suitable for flushing are the fetlock, knee, hock and stifle joints. The joints are washed out with sterile saline, using two large hypodermic needles, one to inject the saline and one to drain the joint. At the end, antibiotic, for example 250 mg gentamicin, is injected into the joint.

See also *Joint-ill of foals* in the section *Infected joints*.

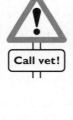

Call vet!

Never fire the skin

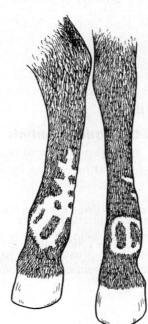

How to treat swollen joints when an animal has been lame for a long time and has old arthritis with new bone around the joint
- Do not rest completely, but give reasonable exercise. Hard work will make the condition worse.
- Make sure the foot is properly shod and balanced.
- Give anti-inflammatory drugs, such as corticosteroids.
- In severe cases, euthanasia is appropriate.
- **Never** burn the skin over the joint. Firing causes great pain to the animal, and does *NOT* help reduce lameness.

5.17 Swelling above fetlock, 'windgall'

These swellings may occur on all four legs. Windgalls are more common in young horses working on hard ground. Windgalls are also seen in older animals, but are not normally important. In adult animals, when there is no lameness and the swelling is not hot, windgalls are a sign of wear of the joint.

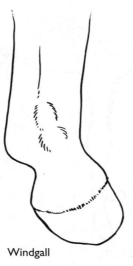

Windgall

What windgalls look like

- Swelling above the fetlocks, often on the inside and outside of the leg.
- Pain and lameness may occur if there is a new injury.

How to treat windgalls

- Stop younger horses from working and rest them.
- Windgalls of older animals do not require treatment when there is no heat or lameness.
- If there is heat, rest the animal.
- If the fetlock joint is very hot or painful, there may be more serious joint disease than windgall. Then treat according to how severe the lameness is, as in the section *Treatment of swollen joints*.

Prevention of more serious problems

Windgalls occur when young horses are made to work on hard ground. If these swellings occur, stop working the animal until there is no more heat in the joint, or else more serious damage to that part of the leg is likely.

5.18 Infected joints

A. Infected joints of adult animals

Infected joints are hot and painful and may discharge pus. Usually infection follows a penetrating wound, for example from a thorn or piece of wire.

How to treat infected joints of adults

Antibiotic injections may help, at least temporarily. The only permanent cure is usually by flushing the joints to wash out all the infection. See the section *Treatment of swollen joints*.

B. Joint-ill of foals

Sometimes all the joints on a foal's leg swell due to infection carried around the body in the blood. Infection can get into the blood through the umbilical cord soon after birth.

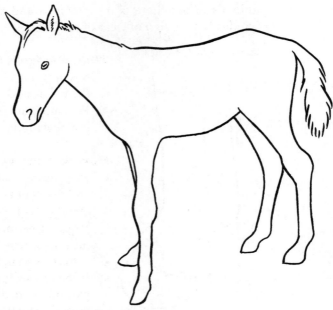

What joint-ill looks like

- Pain and stiffness,
- an awkward walk,
- the foal may be weak and not interested in suckling the mare.

How to prevent joint-ill

Make sure that the area where a mare will give birth is clean, not covered with dung or dirty bedding. Put iodine on the umbilical cord of the foal (see the section *Care of newborn foals*).

How to treat joint-ill

- Give injections of broad-spectrum antibiotics (e.g. penicillin with gentamicin) daily and continue for two weeks after the swellings in the joints have gone down.
- Treatment is not always successful. If the foal does not respond, it is better to kill it humanely (see the chapter *How to shoot a horse*) rather than prolong its pain.

5.19 Hock joint swellings

The hock joint is complex. At the top it moves like a hinge, while at the bottom the joint acts as a 'shock absorber'. Hock joint swellings are more common in animals that pull carts or carriages on hard roads.

Hock joint swellings are called 'spavin'. These swellings may feel soft and fluid or may be bony.

Three other kinds of hock swellings (curb, thoroughpin and slipped flexor tendon) are caused by tendon and ligament injuries.

There is also a fluid swelling under the skin called capped hock.

A.   Fluid swelling of the hock joint ('bog spavin')

Bog spavin refers to the fluid swellings that follow a sprain of the hock joint.

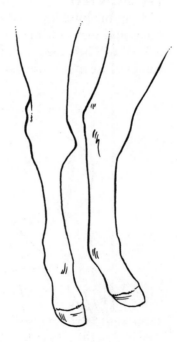

What bog spavin looks like
- Soft, fluid swellings that are found:
  - at the inside front aspect of the joint, and
  - just in front of the point of the hock on either side of the joint.
- The animal is lame and there is heat and pain if the injury is new.
- Bog spavin sometimes develops slowly without heat or pain.

How to prevent bog spavin
Avoid over-working the animal on hard roads.

How to treat bog spavin
- Cool the joint with cold water from a hose or with a bag of ice.
- Rest the animal completely to give the joint a chance to heal.
- Sometimes pain is treated with an anti-inflammatory drug like phenylbutazone, but this may make the horse use the joint too much too soon and so delay healing.

B. Bony swelling on inside of hock ('bone spavin')

This is an example of new bone formation after arthritis. Bone spavin can develop after work on hard roads. The majority of older working horses develop some new bone inside the hock.

What bone spavin looks like

Lameness is worse when the animal first starts trotting. Later in the working day, the animal tends to be less lame.

THE SPAVIN TEST

Pick up the hind leg, hold it with the hock bent for at least 30 seconds, and then trot the animal as soon as the foot is released. The animal will become much lamer if it has spavin. However, this test can produce more lameness with causes other than spavin.

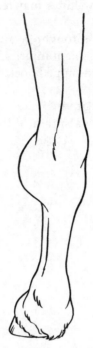

Severe bone spavin.
It may be much
smaller than this.

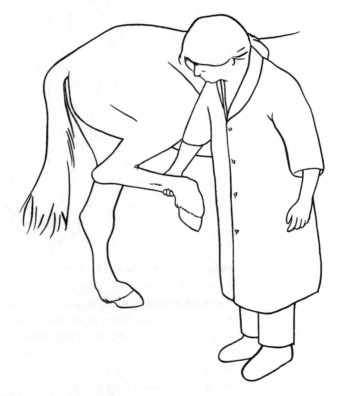

How to prevent bone spavin

- Avoid excessive work on hard roads.
- Reduce the amount of work the animal is asked to do, for example, do not put as many passengers in the *tonga*.

How to treat bone spavin

- Give a little regular exercise. Complete rest is not appropriate.
- Treat with an anti-inflammatory drug like phenylbutazone.

When the horse goes back to work, it may become lame again. On the other hand, more new bone formation due to more work may fix the joint and then the animal can become more sound.

C. Hock ligament injury, 'curb'

'Curb' is an injury to a ligament that runs from the back of the point of the hock down to the top of the cannon bone. An old injury to this ligament can result in a bony lump just below the hock.

What curb looks like
- Some lameness occurs when the injury is new, but the animal is not usually very lame.
- The injury is seen from the side and can be felt.

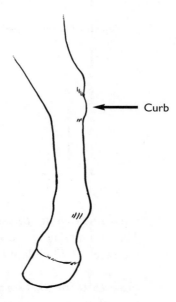

Curb

How to prevent curb
Curb is more common when horses are worked too young or worked too much. Avoid over-working horses, especially young ones.

How to treat curb
- Apply cold water (use a hosepipe if possible) for five minutes every few hours for the first week.
- Give complete rest for two weeks, and then (if there is no sign of lameness) return the animal to light work.

D. Slipped flexor tendon

The support around the tendon is injured in slipped flexor tendon. This support normally keeps the flexor tendon in the right place, over the point of the hock at the back of the leg. (This flexor tendon is not the Achilles tendon which attaches to the hock, it is a tendon that runs over the point of the hock and joins on to bone lower down the leg.) When the support is damaged, the tendon slips round to the side of the hock, usually to the outside.

What slipped flexor tendon looks like
- Pain, swelling and lameness.
- At first you may be able to feel the tendon slipped round to the side.
- Later, the tendon cannot be felt under the fluid in the swelling.

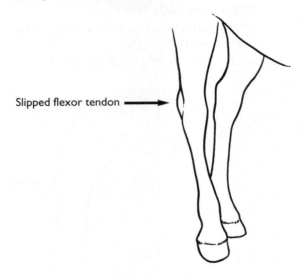

Slipped flexor tendon

How to prevent slipped flexor tendon
The injury usually occurs when a horse is galloping or is in a jumping race. Avoid violent exercise.

How to treat slipped flexor tendon
Complete rest for at least a month. Gradually build up to normal work. Recovery usually takes place, but the injury may occur again.

E.   Thoroughpin
In thoroughpin, there is damage to the sheath around a tendon, which is near the point of the hock. A soft, fluid swelling develops.

What thoroughpin looks like
- A swelling higher than bog spavin is seen in front of the point of the hock.
- The swelling may be on the inside or the outside of the leg.
- If swelling on the outside of the leg is pressed, it bulges on the inside (but not in front of the hock, because the fluid is not within the joint).

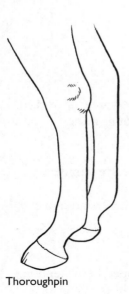

Thoroughpin

How to prevent thoroughpin

Avoid excessive work, because thoroughpin is caused by strain to the sheath of the tendon.

How to treat thoroughpin

- Rest the animal. Only bring it back to work when there is no heat in the area.
- No special treatment is needed unless the tendon has been injured. If so, there may be great pain and a NSAID drug, for example phenylbutazone, should be given.

5.20 Capped elbow and capped hock

These conditions are not really diseases of the joints. The swelling is due to fluid between the skin and the joint.

Capped elbow and capped hock are caused when the elbow or the hock repeatedly knocks a hard surface. Some horses hit their elbow with the heel of the front shoe when they get up or down. This banging from the shoe can eventually lead to capped elbow. Capped hock can occur when the animal often strikes its hock against a wall or partition of a lorry. It can also occur if the animal's hock hits against the front of the cart or vehicle it is pulling.

What capped elbow or hock looks like

- Soft swelling over the point of the hock or elbow.
- The swellings may be painful when they first appear, but do not cause lameness when they are established.

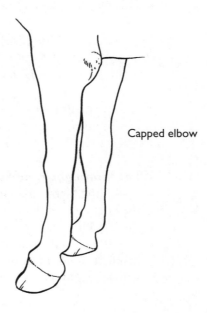

Capped elbow

How to prevent capped elbow or hock

- Make sure the animal has soft bedding. Do not keep a horse or donkey on a hard floor without providing bedding such as straw, wood shavings, torn-up paper strips, or sand.
- Prevent capped elbow by replacing shoes regularly and not letting the heels of the front feet get too long.
- Prevent capped hock by avoiding the possibility of the horse banging its hocks against hard walls or against the cart it is pulling.

How to treat capped elbow or hock

These conditions do not cause lameness, and do not need treatment. Provided that the cause is removed, it is unlikely to get worse.

If the cause is not removed, the swelling may become infected. This is painful and needs treatment with antibiotics. Sometimes antibiotics are not successful in getting rid of the infection.

5.21   Kneecap problems and locked stifle

The horse's kneecap (patella) can get fixed in a position above the joint. When the patella gets stuck in the wrong place, the horse has a 'locked stifle'. This condition is more common in young horses that have not been fed properly and have poor muscle development.

Rarely the kneecap can get into a wrong position on either side of the stifle joint. In this case some of the ligaments that support it must have been damaged.

What locked stifle looks like

- The horse's hind leg is fixed in a straight position.
- This may last for a few seconds or for some hours.

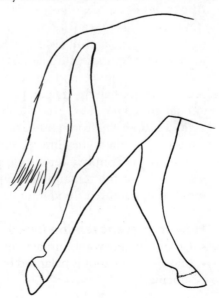

How to prevent locked stifle

Feed young horses well and exercise them regularly. Regular light work helps build muscle around the stifle joint.

How to treat locked stifle

If the kneecap is in the wrong position, it usually clicks back into the correct position when the horse puts weight on that leg.

If the stifle joint remains locked, make the horse walk backwards to force it to put weight on the affected leg.

If the stifle is still locked:

- use a sideline to stretch the leg forwards with a rope from the neck to the fetlock (see *Sideline* in the section *How to restrain horses and donkeys*),
- get another person to push the kneecap up and to the side to attempt to free it.

In cases where the ligaments of the stifle joint have been damaged, a long period of complete rest is needed, perhaps for a year. The horse may never be fully sound.

Tendon injury and other lameness

5.22 Tendon and ligament injuries

This section describes injuries caused by over-stretching of tendons and ligaments. Tendons can also be damaged in deep cuts, especially to the front or back of the legs below the knee. See the section *Leg injuries affecting joints or tendons* in the chapter *How to treat wounds* for advice on tendons damaged in cuts.

About tendons and ligaments

A tendon is like a stretchy rope that connects a muscle to a bone. A ligament is similar, but connects a bone to a bone. There are ligaments that help support the joints in each leg.

Although tendons and ligaments stretch, if over-stretched, they begin to tear. Then the tendon becomes painful and swollen and the animal goes lame. This occurs commonly in animals pulling heavy loads, on both the front and back legs. If seriously over-stretched, a tendon or ligament may break completely.

Tendons heal only after a long period of rest. Healed tendon is less elastic, so the remaining healthy part of the tendon becomes more readily injured. Tendon injuries are best avoided.

How to prevent tendon injury

- Do not subject your animal to extreme work.
- Make sure the foot is balanced by ensuring good trimming and shoeing.

- Regularly feel the animal's tendons and ligaments. If there is pain or heat, rest the animal because more work can make a mild injury severe.
- Take special care with animals pulling or carrying heavy loads to avoid stumbling.

Commonest tendon injuries

The most common site of tendon injury is between the knee and fetlock at the back of the front leg (see the section *How to decide which leg is lame*). The most common ligament injury occurs at the back of the cannon bones, like the tendon injuries. The ligaments are deeper than the tendons.

What ligament or tendon damage looks like

- Sudden lameness.
- Heat, pain and swelling where the structures are injured.

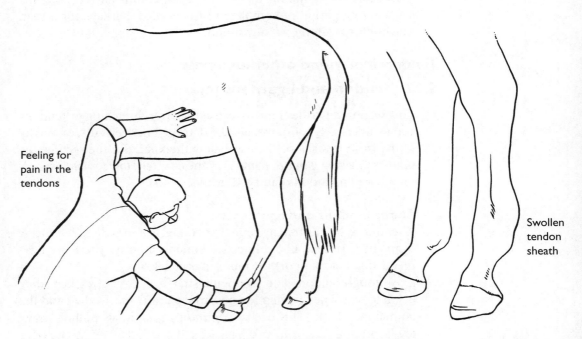

Feeling for pain in the tendons

Swollen tendon sheath

- If a ligament behind the fetlock has broken (ruptured), the fetlock joint drops and is at a different angle, or the toe points up. These cases need a very long period of rest. See the section *Leg injuries affecting joints or tendons* in the chapter *How to treat wounds*.

Management of a tendon injury

FIRST STAGE, FOR THREE OR FOUR WEEKS AFTER THE INJURY

- Pour cold water on the area (use a hose pipe if possible) for five minutes several times a day for the first few days.

- Dry and bandage to support the joint and reduce swelling. Keep bandage over the affected area for three weeks:
  - use cotton wool under the bandage,
  - 'stretchy' support bandages are useful,
  - be careful not to wrap the bandage too tightly around the leg (you should be able to push your finger easily between the skin and the bandage),
  - it is good practice to use a similar bandage to support the opposite leg to the injured one, or it may become injured due to having to carry more weight.
- When the horse is in pain in the first days, give a NSAID drug such as phenylbutazone.
- Complete rest is important at this stage. Keep the animal in a shelter.

SECOND STAGE
- Keep the legs bandaged, and walk the animal around, leading it with a rope, for 30 minutes each day.
- Continue to house the animal when it is not being walked around.

THIRD STAGE, WHEN THERE IS NO LONGER ANY PAIN AND THE ANIMAL IS NOT LAME
- Now the animal should be turned out, no longer kept in the shelter.
- It is very important not to return the animal to hard work for six months.
- During this long third stage, the exercise is gradually increased with more walking. Then after two months, start trotting. If all is going well, cantering can start three months after the injury.

Too much work too soon may delay recovery or cause permanent lameness.

FIRING
Burning the skin over the injury (firing) is *not* helpful. It causes unnecessary suffering and does not help healing. Don't do it.

FUTURE MANAGEMENT OF A WORKING ANIMAL AFTER TENDON INJURY
Tendon injuries can occur repeatedly until the animal becomes more and more lame, and eventually unable to work. The fetlock joint may knuckle over and may develop large windgalls. To avoid this:

- Reduce the load the animal is made to carry or pull.
- Keep the feet balanced and well shod.

Ligament and tendon problems of the hock joint
These are described in the section *Hock joint swellings.*

5.23   Cannon bone problems

A.   Sore shins

This condition affects younger working horses or donkeys that have done a lot of work on hard roads or in sticky mud. It also affects race horses.

What sore shins look like

- A shorter step when trotting.
- The front of the cannon bone on the front leg is very tender when rubbed and may feel warm.

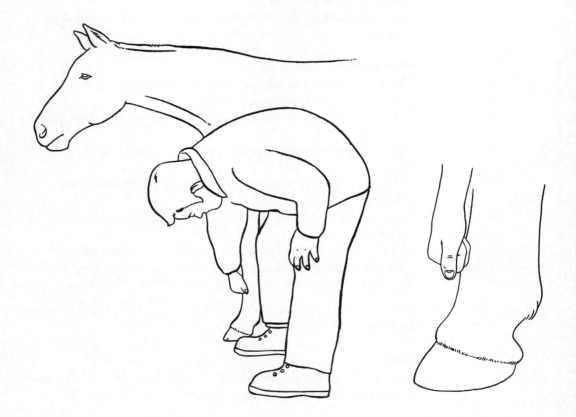

How to prevent sore shins

Do not make young animals work excessively, especially on hard roads.

How to treat sore shins

- Rest for several weeks is essential. Although the soreness may disappear after just a few days rest, it is important not to put the horse straight back into hard work. If you do, there may be permanent damage to the front of the cannon bones, and long-term problems.

- Do not treat by firing. It is cruel and does not help.
- If there is long-term lameness, a NSAID such as phenylbutazone can be used.

B. Splints

'Splint' bone is the common name of two small bones, one on each side of the 'cannon' bone on the front or back leg. The bones are normal, but pain and swelling around them are not.

After injury, eventually abnormal bone develops and this is called 'splints'. It is more common on the front leg, and may develop around the inside or outside splint bone.

Like sore shins, splints usually occur in young horses (less than four years) when they start hard work. They can also develop in older horses that do not have balanced, well-shod feet and in growing horses not fed on a balanced diet.

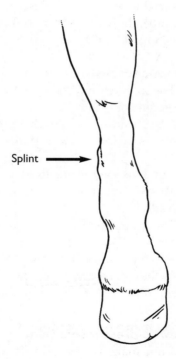

Splint

What splints looks like

- Lameness, especially on rough ground and when trotting down hill.
- Pain when the splint bone area is pressed.
- A swelling develops which eventually becomes hard as new bone forms.

How to prevent splints

- Do not work young horses too hard.
- Feed enough good food to growing horses, especially when about a year old. Growing horses need enough vitamins and minerals in the diet.
- Make sure older horses are shod properly so that the feet are at the right angle.

How to treat splints

Rest completely for three or four weeks until the pain has gone. The new, hard bone will remain. Despite this, usually the horse completely stops being lame. If not, treat with an anti-inflammatory drug such as phenylbutazone.

5.24 Shoulder nerve paralysis, 'sweeney'

In sweeney the muscles over a shoulder become weak following damage to a nerve that runs round the front of the shoulder bone, less than 10 cm above the shoulder joint.

What causes sweeney

- The shoulder hitting something like the side of a door.
- A badly fitting harness that presses on the middle of the shoulder.

What sweeney looks like

- Muscle wastage over the shoulder blade.
- The spine of the shoulder blade is easily felt.
- When the animal takes weight on its foot that side, the point of the shoulder moves away from the body.

Prevention and treatment

Prevent sweeney by making sure that harnesses fit properly. There is no treatment, but rest for a month may lead to recovery. If there is no improvement after this time it is unlikely that the animal will recover. If there is improvement, full recovery may take a year.

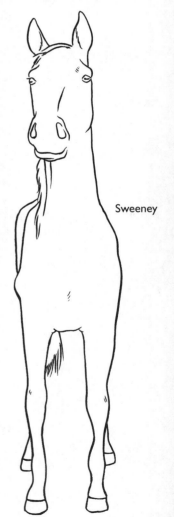

Sweeney

5.25 Tying-up, exertional myopathy

The muscles sometimes become stiff when the animal has a lot of exercise after a period of rest.

What tying-up looks like
- Stiff legs,
- the animal does not want to move or walks with short steps,
- sweating,
- the urine may be dark-coloured.

How to treat tying-up
- Stop working the animal and rest it.
- Give NSAID drugs such as flunixin (Finadyne).
- Do not feed any grain for three days.

6 How to prevent wounds and injuries

6.1 Harnesses

To avoid damaging the skin, harnesses must:

- be cleaned properly,
- be comfortable and made of the right materials (leather is best),
- fit properly,
- be padded,
- have a large enough contact area between the load and the skin to spread the load and prevent heavy rubbing or pressure on a small area of skin.

How to look after leather saddles and tack

Leather needs to be well cared for. Damage by sweat and drying out makes leather hard. Hard leather can injure the skin.

Saddle soap

Saddle soap is useful for regular care of leather saddles and harnesses. To use saddle soap, first wipe down the leather with a damp cloth to remove dirt. Then, get another wet cloth soapy by rubbing it on the saddle soap. Wipe this all over the leather.

How to make saddle soap
1. *Boil a pan of water.*
2. *When it is boiling, add 1 kg of small pieces of washing soap.*
3. *Stir the mixture.*
4. *Skim off and throw away the scum that collects on the surface.*
5. *When the solution becomes thick, add linseed oil. Continue adding and mix thoroughly until it becomes thick and pasty.*
6. *Take it off the heat and cool it. It will look like shoe polish.*

CLEANING LEATHER

Every day, after use:

- Clean leather with a damp cloth or sponge.
- If there is dirt on the leather, use warm water with soap, but do not use a lot of soap because that would remove the oil from the leather and make it hard.

- Scrub off stubborn pieces of dirt.
- Use some horsehair tied in a knot to scrape the leather, or a piece of wood; do not use a sharp tool.
- Do not use detergent and do not use hot water.

OILING LEATHER

Cleaning removes natural oils from leather. Prevent hardening by waxing or oiling when the leather starts to become hard and dry.

What to use to oil leather:

- vegetable oil such as cooking oil,
- animal fat,
- expensive products that can be bought especially for oiling leather.

New, clean, unused engine oil could be used, but is less good. Do not use shoe polish because it does not soften leather.

STORING LEATHER

Store leather harnesses in a dry, airy place. If leather is constantly damp, it may become mouldy. Never leave harnesses on the floor where they can be trodden on and get dirty. Never leave leather in hot sun where it will dry out rapidly.

Materials for making harnesses

As a general principle, only put materials next to an animal's skin that you would have against yours.

GOOD MATERIALS FOR HARNESS PARTS THAT CONTACT THE ANIMAL'S SKIN

- Natural products, like leather and cotton.
- Canvas and synthetic webbing are useful alternatives to leather, but be sure these materials are not abrasive.

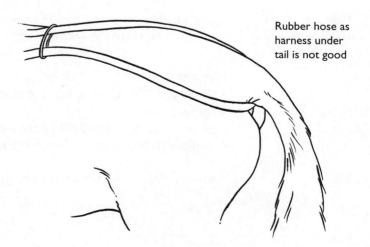

Rubber hose as harness under tail is not good

POOR MATERIALS FOR HARNESS PARTS THAT CONTACT
THE ANIMAL'S SKIN

- Artificial materials, like tyre rubber and nylon rope.
- Wire, thin rope, string and chains should never be against the skin as they are likely to cause injury. There must be enough padding between the skin and these materials if they are components of the harness.
- It is best not to use wire and string for harnesses as they usually soon wear through the padding and can then damage the skin.

Hobbles

Avoid tying a horse or donkey by the leg or foot. Ropes can injure the skin in the hollow of the heel. Tie its head, using a head collar and quick-release knot (see the section *How to tie useful knots*).

If an animal must be hobbled to stop it from running away, the rope around the leg should be tied below the fetlock. (See the section *Checking more closely for the source of lameness* to find out where the fetlock joint is.) Ropes above the fetlock can damage the tendons under the skin.

Do not use strips of nylon tape, the sort that is used to secure boxes. Although very strong, the edge of the tape can easily cut into the skin and cause injury.

6.2 Bits

The best bits are made of stainless steel or aluminium and have a smooth surface.

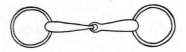 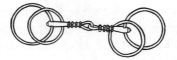 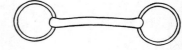

A kind bit that does not injure the mouth

Bits with projections like this are not necessary and cause injury

Another kind bit that does not injure if properly fitted

Bits not to use

- Avoid bits with spurs or parts projecting out. These harsh bits are not necessary.
- Avoid sharp bits because they can injure the angle of the lips.
- Avoid iron bits, because they may rust and get sharp edges.

Do not place the bit too tightly in the mouth.

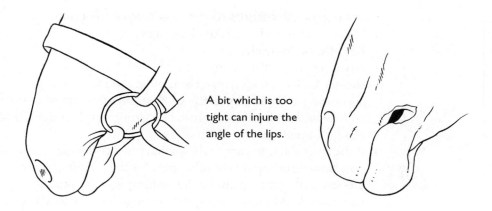

A bit which is too tight can injure the angle of the lips.

6.3 Pack animals

Padding for pack animals

When a working animal carries pack loads or panniers hung over its back, it is essential that there is padding between the load and the animal to protect the skin from rubbing injuries. Thin animals need thicker padding.

LOOKING AFTER COTTON OR WOOLLEN PADDING

Wash saddle cloths or *numnahs* in the same way that you wash your own clothing. Dry well in the sun before putting back on a horse or donkey.

LAYERS OF PADDING

Usually, there are three parts to the equipment put on the back of a pack animal: the padding layer, then a cushioning layer and then the saddle or container for the load.

The padding next to the skin

Several layers of cotton material next to the skin is ideal. This layer should be made of material that can be washed. Cotton is suitable because it is soft for protection and absorbs sweat. The padding layer next to the skin should be replaced or washed regularly.

The next layer, the cushioning layer

This layer is usually not easy to wash. Locally made padding (made from old blankets) is good. A folded blanket or a padded sack can be used instead. With the latter it is important to sew the bag into sections to prevent the straw or other filling from falling to one end.

The saddle or holder for whatever is to be carried sits on the padding.

HOW TO REDUCE WOUNDS TO THE SKIN UNDER THE LOAD

- Make sure the padding is thick enough.
- Keep the padding clean.
- Dry it before putting it on.
- Hessian or jute sacking material is often used for making harnessing and padding. If the sacking has been soaked in sweat and allowed to dry, it can become very rough and scratchy. If so, wash it or replace it.
- If the animal has to carry a dirty load, put a cotton sheet over the skin before putting on the other parts of the padding to prevent dirt and grit getting between the padding and the skin.
- Padding should protect the spine. Arrange it so the load presses each side of the back bone, and not on the ridge of the spine itself.

Loading

HOW MUCH LOAD TO PUT ON

Excessive workloads cause injury to the skin, joint problems and shorten an animal's working life. Overloading a cart or *tonga* may bring more income today, but will reduce it in future, because a new horse must be paid for.

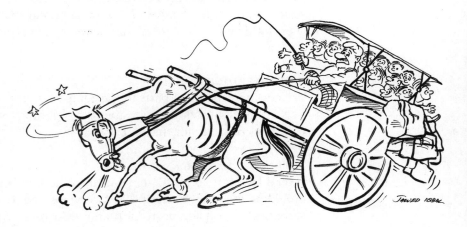

A pack animal can safely carry a third to a half of its own weight for several hours if it is in reasonable condition, that is, about 40 kg of load per 100 kg of its body weight. This means that an appropriate load for a typical donkey to carry for a few hours is approximately 50–100 kg. Reduce this if the load will be carried all day.

See the section *How to estimate body weight*, then estimate suitable loads by working out what is one third of this amount.

HOW TO POSITION THE LOAD

Good positioning of the load reduces injuries to the animal's skin. It also makes best use of the animal's energy, as an unbalanced load requires more energy to transport than a balanced load.

For pack-saddles or panniers make sure that:

- the load is put over the shoulders just behind the withers, and
- the load is distributed evenly on each side of the animal to ensure a balanced load and to stop the load from slipping over to one side.

HOW TO SECURE THE LOAD

The load must be properly secured. For light loads, use rubber strips cut from the inner tubes of car or lorry tyres. These strips are stretchy, which helps fix the load.

For heavier loads, use ropes to fasten them to the saddle. Ropes should be tied with knots that are both secure and able to be undone quickly if the animal needs to be freed from the load, for example, if it falls. See the section *How to tie useful knots*.

Breeching and breast straps

BREECHING STRAP FOR ANIMALS PULLING CARTS OR TONGAS

The breeching is the part of the harness that comes around the back end of the animal. Without one, the other parts of the harness slide forward when the animal stops or goes down hill. These parts of the harness can cause injuries to the skin, for example, above the shoulders or behind the front legs.

BREAST STRAP AND BREECHING STRAP FOR PACK ANIMALS

If hills are to be encountered on the journey the load must be secured at the front and back. To do this, a breast strap is used at the front. At the back, a breeching rope is passed around the upper legs of the animal.

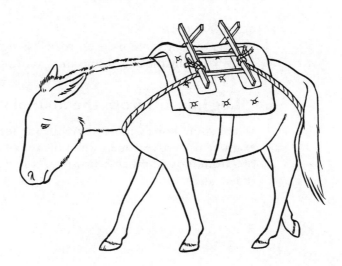

BALANCING THE LOAD ON A TWO-WHEEL CART

Balance the load on a two-wheel cart. Make sure the load is balanced over the wheels so there is no upward lift by the shafts.

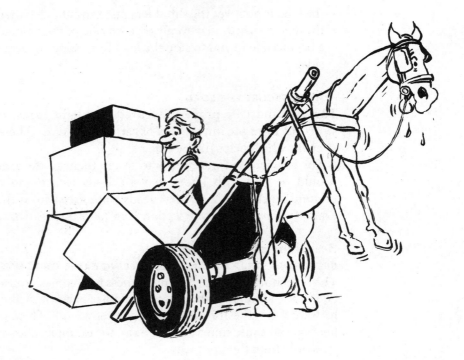

Design features of carts and wagons

NOT TOO HEAVY

Ideally, carts for a single donkey should be made of strong, light materials and weigh no more than 100 kg. The cart should have a load capacity of 250–350 kg.

BE SEEN AT NIGHT

If carts or *tongas* are used on roads at night, make them easier to see by painting the back white and by fitting large reflectors.

6.4   Leg injuries from the animal kicking itself

When some horses move they hit one leg with another leg. One example is 'over-reaching', when the toe of a back foot hits the heel of a front foot. Another is 'brushing', when a foot hits the leg on the other side.

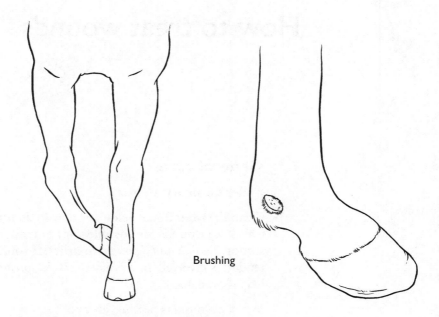

Brushing

How to prevent injuries from one leg interfering with another

Sometimes these injuries occur because the shoeing is not correct. Check that the shoes are properly fitted. It may be possible to fit a special shoe with the part of the shoe that hits the other leg set back, so that metal cannot hit against the other leg.

Injuries from brushing or over-reaching can be prevented with a piece of rubber inner tube stitched in place. For brushing, a roll of cloth can be effective.

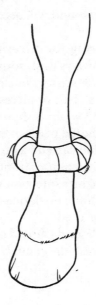

7   How to treat wounds

7.1   General care

Just after the injury, always:

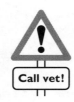

- Clean the wound (see below for how to do this).
- Check leg wounds for possible joint or tendon injury (see the section *Tendon and ligament injuries*). If you think a joint or tendon is involved, immediately call for professional veterinary help if available.

While a wound is healing, always:

- Rest the animal until healing is complete, so that work does not make the wound worse.
- Remove the cause of the wound, for example, by repairing a badly fitting harness.

7.2   How to care for a fresh wound

It is important to wash a wound. If you do not, it is more likely that the wound will become infected and then healing may be delayed.

Caring for a fresh wound
- Always wash your hands before touching a wound.
- Use scissors to clip hair from around the edge of the wound. Pick any hair or pieces of dirt or small stones out of the wound.
- All wounds should be washed. Use very clean water. The water should be clean enough to drink, or boil and cool it.
- You can add a little salt, one teaspoonful of salt to 500 ml water.
- Do not use strong disinfectants on the wound. Few chemicals reduce infection without damaging the wound.
- Dilute povidone-iodine made specially for washing wounds can be used.
- Wounds should be washed twice daily for at least five minutes. To wash the wound, you can:

◦ either pour slowly,

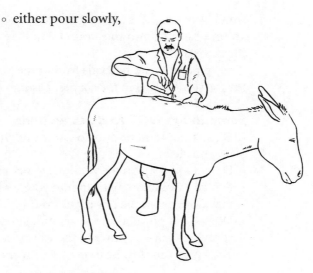

◦ or use a hose pipe,

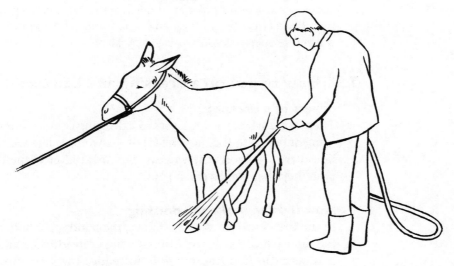

◦ or use a syringe to squirt water to wash it (the ideal pressure comes from squirting water from a 30 ml syringe through an 18 g needle),
◦ or use a large wad of very wet cotton and soak the wound.

- Allow it to dry in air, while keeping flies away.
- Cover the wound with a dressing (see the next section, *How to put on a dressing and bandage*) unless the wound is small.

Fly repellent

Flies are attracted by the smell of a wound. Flies can bring infection, which slows down healing.

You can make fly repellent by mixing a large spoonful of kerosene (paraffin) in a bucket containing 3 litres of water. Mix it well so that small droplets of kerosene form in the water. Put this mixture around but not into the wound. Flies are kept away by the smell of the kerosene.

Fly repellents can be made from some plants, such as the neem tree. See the section *Flies* in the chapter *Diseases and parasites of the skin*.

Some things NOT to do to wounds

- Do not put mud or dung on a wound. It is important to keep the wound clean.
- Do not use soap on the wound. Do not put anything in the wound that you would not like put into your own eye. Anything that hurts may do harm to the raw edges from which the wound will heal.
- Do not put powder on the wound. Do not spray with a 'purple spray' aerosol except when the wound is on or under the hoof. The spray can slow healing of skin wounds.

Only when water is not available, for example when pack animals are at work, wound powder or aerosol can be used to give a temporary protection from flies and infection. The wound should be washed properly as soon as is practical.

7.3 How to put on a dressing and bandage

Layers of a dressing

There are normally three layers to a dressing over a wound. The first is in contact with the raw surface of the wound. The second absorbs liquid and cushions the wound. The third layer is the bandage to hold the other two layers in place.

How tight to make the dressing

In the first few days after the injury, the bandage should not be tied too tightly. Make sure you can put a finger inside the bandage. Later, it is better to tie it more tightly to reduce the formation of excess granulation tissue or proud flesh.

How to put on a bandage

A bandage is wrapped around the leg over the contact and absorbing layers. The bandage has to be tight enough not to slip down, but not so tight that it stops blood flowing in the leg. The pictures on the page overleaf show how to wrap the bandage around the leg.

The hock and the knee can be bandaged in a similar way. Be sure to use plenty of padding over bony joints.

Layers of dressing and examples of materials

Layer of dressing	Example materials
The first layer, in contact with the injury This layer needs to be perfectly clean, non-sticky and able to let liquid from the wound pass through it to the next layer	**Cotton gauze or cotton wool** (clean, unspun cotton): this tends to stick to the wound; it is difficult to remove without causing damage to the healing surface and pain.
	Gauze with petroleum jelly (Vaseline) or **Tulle**: this sticks less than cotton; it can be bought from pharmacies, usually in flat tins.
	Specially made pads (e.g. Melolin) with a shiny, non-stick surface to put against the wound: these are best because they do not stick, do not leave any bits in the wound when removed, are perfectly clean and are good at keeping the wound dry.
The second layer, the padding layer This layer needs to be very clean, absorbent and soft.	**Cotton wool**: this is available in most countries and is reasonably cheap.
	Disposable nappies (diapers): these are expensive, but very good at absorbing liquid from big wounds in the first days after injury.
	Towelling cloth: this is absorbent, but tends to stick; use it if you do not have alternative materials.
The third layer, the bandage layer This layer holds the first two in place. The material needs to be clean, strong and in a long strip to wind around the leg or tail.	**Crepe bandage**: this is available from pharmacies and clinics.
	Strips of cotton cloth cut from old bed-sheets or clothes: as good as bandages bought from shops, but make sure the cloth is clean.
	Sticky and/or stretchy rolls, for example, Elastoplast: these materials are very useful, but expensive and difficult to buy in many countries; the main advantage is that these types are best at stopping the first two layers slipping down the leg.

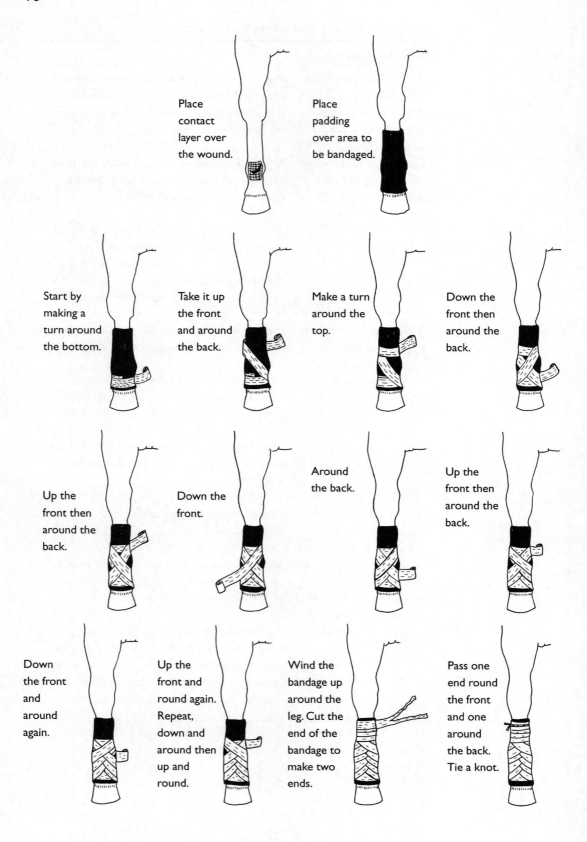

Place contact layer over the wound.

Place padding over area to be bandaged.

Start by making a turn around the bottom.

Take it up the front and around the back.

Make a turn around the top.

Down the front then around the back.

Up the front then around the back.

Down the front.

Around the back.

Up the front then around the back.

Down the front and around again.

Up the front and round again. Repeat, down and around then up and round.

Wind the bandage up around the leg. Cut the end of the bandage to make two ends.

Pass one end round the front and one around the back. Tie a knot.

7.4 How to treat cuts and grazes and skin tears

Grazes and small wounds

Clean the wound as described above. For most wounds, no more treatment is needed. Most small wounds do not need to be bandaged and heal faster without being covered.

Simple cuts

If not suitable for stitching, treat by cleaning and dressing (bandaging) the wound as described above. Some new cuts are suitable for stitching. See the section *How to stitch a cut*.

Skin tears

- Clean the wound carefully.
- Make sure there is no dirt trapped under the flap of skin.
- The edges of tears with small flaps can sometimes be stitched back together, especially if the wound is on the animal's head or body and the wound is fresh.
- If a flap of skin has become dry and dead, it is usually best to cut it off using perfectly clean scissors or a sharp knife, like a razor blade.
- Keep the wound clean, by washing it as for other wounds.
- Cover the wound with a dressing if you can. Transparent tape (e.g. Sellotape) can be used to hold a clean dressing over a wound on the body or head where it cannot be bandaged.

7.5 How to stitch a cut

Cuts suitable for stitching

- Wounds on the head or body,
- fresh cuts, less than four hours old,
- deep, clean cuts where the skin edges are not grazed or torn,
- wounds which gape open.

Cuts that should not be stitched

- Wounds on the lower legs,
- old wounds, more than eight hours old,
- dirty wounds,
- dog bite wounds,
- puncture wounds.

Old wounds and bite wounds can sometimes be stitched after they have been properly cleaned, and if the skin edges are freshened, that is, cut back to make fresh, new edges.

Equipment used for stitching

- Local anaesthetic

  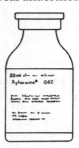

  See list of medicines at the back of the book

- Syringe and hypodermic needle

  The needle should be of a size suitable for subcutaneous injection, for example, 21 or 23 gauge (see the section How to give injections*)*

- Needle

  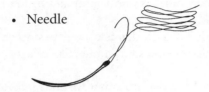

  A sewing needle will do, but it is easier with a vet's needle or strong cobbler's needle

- Thread

  Preferably nylon (thin, mono-filament nylon fishing line is ideal) or silk. Cotton is not ideal as it acts like a wick and then attracts dirt when it is wet

- Scissors

  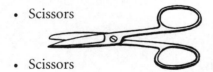

  To cut hair around the wound. A razor blade or scalpel blade could be used instead

- Scissors

  A clean pair to snip the thread

- Soap and boiled water

  To wash hands

- Cotton wool

  Or very clean cloth, preferably boiled and then dried

- Antiseptic solution in a bowl to clean the wound

  See the section How to care for a fresh wound *for suitable antiseptics*

Preparation

- If the needle, thread and scissors are not sterilized and packed (see the section *How to sterilize equipment*), boil them in a pan of water for 10 minutes, then pour off the water and allow time for them to cool.
- Wash your hands.
- Clip or shave hair around the skin edges if the cut is in a hairy place.
- Wash the wound as described in the section *How to care for a fresh wound*.

Anaesthetic

If you have local anaesthetic solution for injection, inject it around the wound.

- Inject 0.5 ml in each place. It seems less painful for the animal to inject from inside the wound.

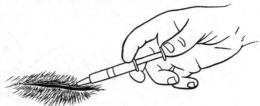

- Wait a few minutes.
- Before starting to stitch, test that the anaesthetic has worked by pricking around the wound with a needle. The horse should not feel the pricking.

Threading the needle

- Wash your hands again using new, clean water and soap or antiseptic.
- If you are using nylon thread, which is slippery, thread the needle twice. This helps to stop the thread coming out of the needle as the needle is pulled through.

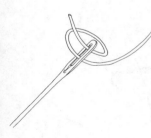

Putting in stitches

- Turn the edges of the skin out rather than in when pushing the needle through so that when the stitch is tightened the raw undersides of the skin touch.
- If the wound bleeds and this obscures your view, press and hold very clean cotton or very clean cloth on it between stitches.
- Stitch from left to right, if it is a straight cut and you are right-handed.
- With an odd-shaped wound, start by putting a stitch in the middle of the wound.

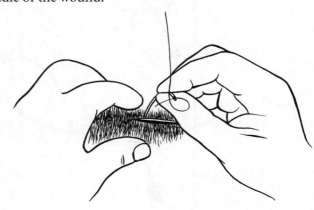

Tying the knot

- Do *not* pull the thread tight; it should just bring the edges of the skin together.

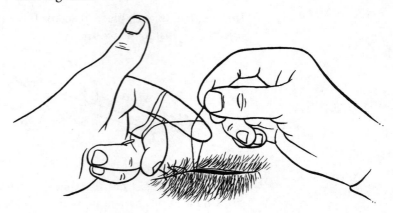

- Tie the knot with a double turn first and then two or more single turns.
- Nylon thread is slippery and needs extra tying.

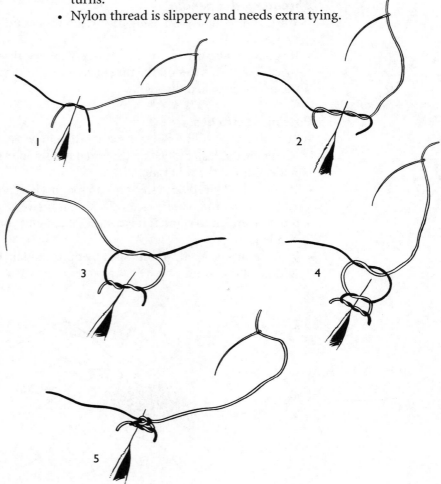

- Cut the thread so that the ends are quite long, at least 1 cm. This gives you more to hold when taking stitches out.

Healing

There may be a few drops of bloody discharge from the wound for the first two days. If the wound swells and looks infected (e.g. discharging pus, or smelling or attracting many flies) take the lower stitches out immediately. Wash the wound and leave it open to heal. Treat it as an infected wound (see the section *Infected wounds*).

Taking out stitches

Stitches normally need to be removed after 10 days.

- Cut the thread on one side of the knot on each stitch.
- Then pull the knot to pull out the stitch.

Cutting the thread does not hurt, but pulling a stitch out can cause some pain which could make the animal react aggressively. So cut all the stitches first and then pull the knots quickly one by one.

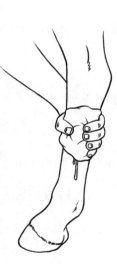

7.6 Severe bleeding

First, *very* firmly hold a thick layer of cotton wool or clean cloth on the wound for five minutes.

Then, if the severely bleeding wound is on a leg where it can be bandaged, apply a pressure bandage.

How to apply a pressure bandage

- Put a thick layer of cotton wool or cloth on the wound and right around the leg. It must be thick, at least 4 cm of cotton.
- Bind strips of cloth tightly over it.

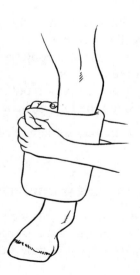
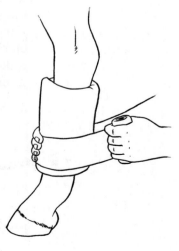

- Leave the pressure bandage on for at least two hours and for up to 12 hours. If the bleeding starts again when the bandage is removed, apply another pressure bandage. If the bleeding has stopped, treat as an ordinary fresh wound.

7.7 Pressure sores

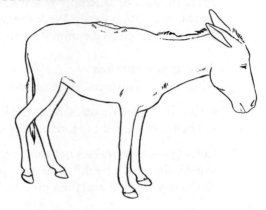

These wounds take a long time to heal, typically two to three months.

How to treat pressure sores
- For the first three or four days, clean the sore twice daily until it looks pink and healthy. See the section *How to care for a fresh wound*.
- Then apply cream like zinc oxide ointment or petroleum jelly each day. The cream helps to keep the wound moist so it does not dry and crack. It also acts as a barrier to infection.
- If possible, do not make the animal carry a load until the sore has healed.
- It is essential to think about what caused the injury and how to remove the cause. For example:
  ○ if the animal is too thin and bony, try to buy more food for it or allow it more time to eat, or
  ○ if the padding under the pack is old and sweaty, wash it, or
  ○ if the padding is not thick enough, make more padding.

See the section *Pack animals* for advice on how to prevent pressure sores.

7.8 Proud flesh, excess granulation tissue

This is a complication of wound healing that occurs on the lower parts of horses' and donkeys' legs. It is more common in horses.

Proud flesh occurs when the pink or red healing tissue in the

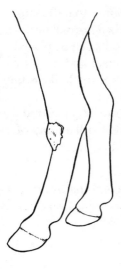

middle of a wound grows faster than the skin edges around the wound. This lump of tissue will get bigger and bigger unless the skin can grow over it.

What causes proud flesh

- Infection of the wound,
- movement of the edges of the wound, for example, because the wound is over a joint.

How to treat proud flesh

MAKE SURE THAT THE WOUND IS VERY CLEAN

- Wash the wound as described in the the section *How to care for a fresh wound*.
- It may be useful to wash the wound with a solution of antibiotic powder, for example, ampicillin. In some countries, only veterinarians and medical workers can buy ampicillin, but in many countries, pharmacies sell ampicillin capsules to anybody. The capsules are broken open so the powder can be mixed with very clean water (boiled and then allowed to cool).

USE A CORTICOSTEROID CREAM

- Apply the cream to the proud flesh twice daily.
- Do not put cream on the skin edges, but only on the lump of red tissue.

Examples of corticosteroid creams are listed at the back of the book.

Get trained helper!

CUT IT OFF AND APPLY PRESSURE BANDAGE

- For safety, if operating on a back leg, put on sidelines (see the section *How to restrain horses and donkeys*).
- Use a sharp knife like a razor blade. Cut the proud tissue back to skin level. This tissue does not have any nerves, so it will not hurt the horse to cut it. If you cut the skin, it hurts.
- It will always bleed a lot, but there is rarely any infection. If you start cutting at the bottom of the wound and work up, it is easier to see what you are doing. If you start at the top of the wound, blood tends to run down into the place where you are cutting.
- After cutting, bandage as described in the sections *Severe bleeding* and *How to put on a dressing and bandage*. Change the dressing every two or three days.
- The skin edges should start to grow in from the sides of the wound. If the proud tissue grows back faster, carefully cut it back again, this time to about 0.5 cm below the skin level, and bandage again.

OLDER TREATMENTS WITH CAUSTIC CHEMICALS

- It is possible to use copper sulphate or magnesium sulphate

(Epsom salts) to kill the proud flesh. The problem is that the same chemicals can kill the skin edges and so slow down normal healing.

- Copper sulphate crystals or a paste of Epsom salts can be placed on the centre of the proud flesh, bandaged in place and left for a few days. Epsom salts will produce an unpleasant smell like rotten eggs.
- Then remove the dressing and look at the wound. If the proud flesh is reduced, treat as a fresh wound. If there is still a lump of proud flesh, repeat the chemical treatment, but change the dressing after one day.

Proud flesh can take a long time to cure. A combination of cutting, using a chemical and using cream may work best. Every case is different.

7.9 Infected wounds

Infected wounds may smell, discharge pus and attract a lot of flies. The animal may be unwell and may have stopped eating.

How to treat old, infected wounds
- Wash the wound with a hosepipe or use several buckets full of water. Use plenty of water.
- Apply some antiseptic to the wound by squirting with a syringe or with cotton wool, as described in the section *How to care for a fresh wound*.

Suitable antiseptics

Add iodine to the water to turn it the colour of very weak tea.
   If you do not have iodine, less good, but still useful alternatives are:
- *add 2 teaspoonfuls of salt to 1 litre of water, or*
- *a pinch of crystals of potassium permanganate (to make a purple solution), or*
- *a pinch of crystals of mercurochrome (to make a red solution).*

- Let the wound dry and apply antibiotic ointment (not powder).

Treatment if the horse is sick
- If the infection is severe, the animal's behaviour may become dull or depressed and it may stop eating. It may be ill because infection or toxins (poisons caused by the infection) have spread from the wound. A sick animal should be injected with antibiotic, such as long-acting penicillin.
- If there is no improvement in the animal after two days, or sooner, consult a veterinarian if possible.

7.10 Fly-blown wounds, screw worm

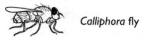

Calliphora fly

Maggots often infest animal wounds, especially when the wound is infected, because the smell of the infection attracts flies. Flies lay eggs that hatch into maggots and burrow into the wound. The maggots may go deep into the flesh and cause the skin to lift off.

Screw worm

Screw worm disease is the infestation of a wound with a particularly damaging type of maggot. Screw worms are most common in tropical, humid climates. In many countries, suspected infections should be reported to the veterinary authorities.

What screw worm disease looks like
- Screw worms burrow more deeply than the maggots of other flies.
- A foul-smelling brown fluid pours from the wound and this attracts more flies.
- Maggots can soon eat large areas of tissue.

How to prevent maggots from infesting wounds
- Keep wounds clean.
- Use a fly repellent (see the section *How to care for a fresh wound* above) around the wound.
- Burn or bury dead bodies where flies breed.

How to treat wounds with maggots
- Clip the hair away from the wound and any tracks where the maggots are burrowing.
- Soak cotton wool in a chemical that kills the maggots. Hold it on the wound for a few minutes.

> Chemicals and mixtures to kill maggots
> - *Most chemicals used to control ticks (see the section* Ticks) *are effective against maggots. Usually these chemicals must be mixed with water before use. Carefully follow instructions on the label.*
> - *Mix kerosene or turpentine with boric acid powder and spread it on the fly-blown wound.*
> - *Chloroform, but be careful not to breathe in the fumes of this chemical.*

- A few drops of ivermectin for injection (sold for cattle) can be squirted directly on to the wound. This kills the maggots rapidly.
- Pick the maggots out of the wound.
- Wash the wound.

- Dry the wound with clean cloth or cotton wool.
- Apply antiseptic ointment, such as zinc oxide.
- Repeat these steps every day until the wound is free of maggots and infection.
- If the wound was a puncture wound, and maggots have made tracks under the skin, it may be necessary to cut off the skin over these maggot tracks.

7.11 Leg injuries affecting joints or tendons

Injuries to tendons caused by over-stretching them in work are described in the *Lameness* chapter in the section *Tendon and ligament injuries*. Tendons can also be damaged by deep cuts. They take months to heal. If you suspect that joints or tendons are involved in a wound, get advice from a veterinarian if possible.

How to recognize tendon involvement
Look closely at the angle of the joints of the foot. The normal angle is shown in the section *Normal feet and legs*. Be suspicious of damage to the tendons at the back of the leg if the angle of the pastern joint has dropped. When tendons above the back of the foot are damaged, the fetlock joint may have a different angle.

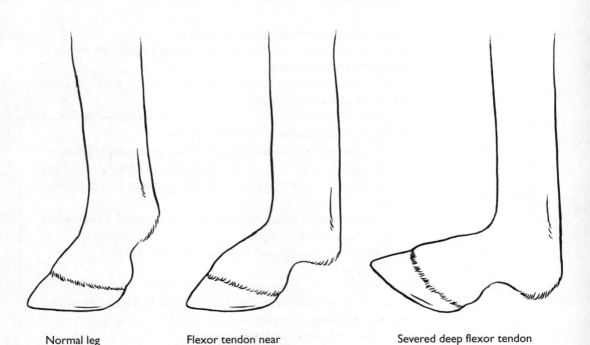

Normal leg

Flexor tendon near the surface cut

Severed deep flexor tendon

The tendons on the front of the leg (extensor tendons) can be injured when there is a wound to the front of the cannon. Damage is not always seen immediately. It can occur a week or two later, if the blood supply to the tendons had been damaged by the original injury.

HOW TO TREAT INJURY TO THE TENDONS
- Complete rest until the swelling goes down.
- Hose the painful, swollen part of the leg with cold water, or put cloths soaked in cold water on the leg. Do this several times a day for three days.
- Dry the leg, and bandage to reduce the swelling.
- Give pain relief with a NSAID drug. See list at the back of the book.
- Animals with cut tendons should be given antibiotic injections for at least seven days. If the skin is not cut, do not give antibiotics.

Tendons take *at least six weeks* to repair properly, depending on how severe the injury was. It is necessary to stop work and completely rest the animal for a month and then give light exercise for two weeks. Six weeks after the injury, the animal may do light work for several months. If you start to work the animal hard too soon, it will probably be lame for much longer.

Injuries affecting a joint
It is important to recognize the possibility of joint injury, because if infection starts in a joint it can result in permanent lameness. Deep wounds near a joint sometimes puncture the joint itself.

WHAT JOINT INJURY LOOKS LIKE
Although there is always some fluid (serum) which drips out of any wound as it begins to heal, be suspicious that a joint is damaged if you see leakage of clear liquid. More fluid may leak when the joint is bent.

HOW TO TREAT INJURY TO JOINTS
- Clean the wound. See the section *How to care for a fresh wound*.
- Give antibiotic injections for five days. See the section *Infected joints* in the *Lameness* chapter.

7.12 Broken bones

Bones can break in road accidents or from a kick by another horse or during strenuous exercise such as jumping. Sometimes a mare treads on her foal and breaks its leg.

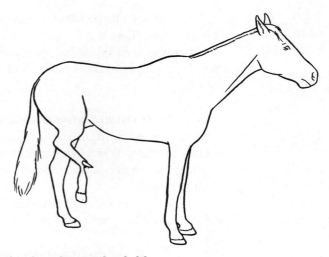

What broken bones look like

- A horse with a fracture is usually in great pain and will not put any weight at all on the affected leg.
- The leg may have a different shape, with a bend in it where there is not a joint.
- There may be a large swelling due to bleeding inside the leg.
- The end of a broken bone may stick out of a wound in the skin.
- A broken bone high up in the leg, for example on the hind leg between the hip and stifle joint, can be difficult to see, because there is a lot of muscle over these bones. If you press your ear to the leg, you might hear the grating sound of the broken end of bone.
- If a bone is broken high up on the front leg, the horse may stand with its elbow dropped, as shown in the picture below.

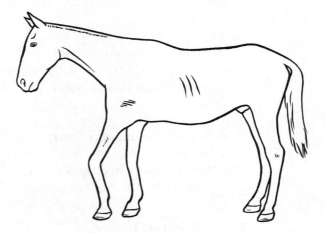

Whether or not to treat broken bones

When a working horse or donkey breaks a bone in its leg, the appropriate action is normally euthanasia. See *How to shoot a horse*.

Euthanasia is also normally recommended for fractures in the legs of foals. However, a young foal or donkey with a fracture low down the leg may have a chance of normal healing, if:

- the fracture is below the knee or hock,
- there is no bone sticking out through the skin, and
- the animal can be rested in a quiet place for several weeks at least while the bone has a chance to heal.

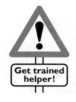

Get trained helper!

If possible, get these cases seen at a veterinary clinic. If treated properly with a cast, this kind of fracture in a donkey or foal may heal. If no professional advice is available, consult a local bone-setter for advice on how to support the injury with splints.

7.13 Burns

How to treat burns

- Put cold water on the burnt areas immediately. Continue to pour cold water on the burnt areas for ten minutes. This reduces the damage that the heat will cause.
- Later, if the burn has caused blistering of the skin, apply petroleum jelly (Vaseline) or calamine lotion.
- Apply fly repellent (see the sections *How to care for a fresh wound* and *Flies*)

Euthanasia is recommended if the burning is serious. Euthanasia should be considered if:

- there are severe burns that cause charring of the flesh,
- burns affect more than 20% of the body surface, or
- the animal is unconscious or unable to walk.

7.14 Injury to the head or spine

When the brain or the spinal cord is damaged, the animal may behave in an abnormal way. In some cases the damage is severe and recovery is impossible.

If any of the following signs are seen, there is little possibility of improvement, and therefore euthanasia is recommended:

1 Coma (the animal appears to be asleep, and cannot be made to wake up).
2 All legs are stretched out straight and rigid.
3 The pupils (the black centre part) of both eyes are big, black circles.
4 There are strange patterns of breathing.
5 The horse does not give any response to pain, for example pinching the skin hard in the lower legs.

8 Lumps under the skin

8.1 Different kinds of swellings

Common swellings appearing as lumps under the skin are abscess, rupture, hernia, haematoma, tumour, cyst and oedema.

Different kinds of swellings

Name of swelling	What it is
Abscess	• caused by infection • consists of pus
Rupture, hernia	• often follows injury • some of what is normally inside the belly, for example, abdominal fat or a loop of intestine, comes through a hole in the layers of muscle under the skin and lies under the skin
Blood blister or haematoma	• a swelling containing blood • happens when an injury causes bleeding under the skin
Cyst	• contains fluid from a gland
Growth or tumour	• a growth caused by the rapid division of cells • some tumours seed secondary growths in other parts of the body • other growths just get bigger where they are
Oedema	• caused when fluid accumulates within tissue • can result from an allergic reaction

8.2 Abscess and how to recognize and treat it

It is very important not to mistake a hernia or rupture for an abscess. Because an abscess is a swelling with pus beneath the skin like a very large boil, the aim when treating it is to get the infection (pus) to drain away completely. This may involve 'lancing' or cutting the skin.

Hernias or ruptures are usually below the belly and may contain internal organs like a loop of intestine. Cutting a swelling like this could be disastrous. Be careful.

What a hernia or rupture looks like

- Suspect a hernia or rupture particularly when the swelling is around the testicles or the body wall.
- Feel the swelling carefully. Can you feel a loop of intestine or something else which is not fluid in the swelling? Can you push the contents of the swelling back into the body? If so it is probably a rupture or hernia which may need surgery.

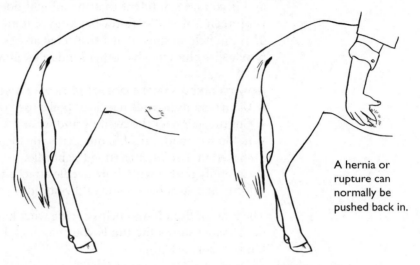

A hernia or rupture can normally be pushed back in.

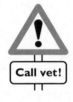

Call vet!

- Do not try to treat a hernia or rupture. Contact a veterinary surgeon.

What an abscess looks like

- Abscesses are usually hot and painful when touched, but hernias and ruptures that have been there for some time often are not painful. Haematoma, oedema, cyst and tumour swellings are not normally painful.
- If it is an abscess there may be a scar on the skin where there was a wound which allowed the infection in.
- Gentle squeezing pressure may cause pus to drip or even burst out if it is 'ripe'.

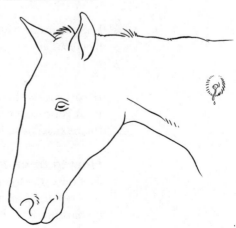

- An abscess is often hotter than the surrounding skin and may be quite painful: the animal may respond when you touch it.
- Because of the infection in an abscess the animal's temperature is often higher than normal.

How to confirm that a swelling is an abscess

If the infection does not burst and discharge the infection naturally and if you are confident that the animal does not have a hernia or rupture, it is useful to find what kind of liquid is inside the swelling. This can help to show that a suspected abscess really is an abscess, or it may give clues to what other kind of swelling it is.

HOW TO TAKE A SAMPLE OF LIQUID FROM A SWELLING

- Use a new, disposable needle or boil a used one for 10 minutes first.
- Cut the hair over the swelling and wash it with soap and water.
- If you have some alcohol or spirit wipe the skin with a cotton pad soaked in it before inserting the needle.
- Carefully push a wide-bore needle attached to a syringe into the lump and suck back some of the liquid.

The kind of fluid found helps decide what kind of swelling it is. The table below shows the fluids you may suck back from the different kinds of soft swellings.

Kinds of fluid found in different types of swellings

Type of swelling	Kind of liquid found in the swelling
Abscess	Abscesses usually contain creamy white, bad-smelling pus; sometimes the pus is bloody
Tumour or growth	Tumours are often solid and it may not be possible to withdraw any fluid
Cyst	Cysts contain fluid (e.g. cysts on the side of the head may contain saliva)
Haematoma or blood blister	Bleeding under the skin causes a haematoma; you may suck back fresh blood or clotted blood and serum, which looks like watery blood

If you sucked back some pus from the swelling, and the other signs fit, it is probably an abscess. Proceed with the treatment described in the next section. If in doubt, get help from a veterinarian if possible.

How to treat an abscess

The best way to ensure that an abscess will drain completely is to get it to ripen, burst and drain naturally. You can encourage this process by bathing it with hot compresses.

HOW TO BATHE AN ABSCESS

- Mix salt or Epsom salts (magnesium sulphate) in water as hot as you can comfortably bear your hands in. Add a teaspoonful of salt in 1 pint or 0.5 litre of water.
- Soak a piece of clean cloth or cotton wool with this solution and hold it on the swelling.
- When the cloth gets cool soak it in the hot solution again.
- Continue for about five minutes.
- Do this at least four times a day.

The skin may soften and break, discharging pus, which usually smells foul. Keep on bathing with salt solution to encourage the drainage to continue so that no pus remains inside when the skin closes and heals.

If the abscess does not burst, it may be necessary to lance it.

HOW TO CUT (LANCE) AN ABSCESS

- Use a very sharp, very clean blade.
- Cut away the hair over the abscess with scissors.
- Wash the skin with soap and water.
- Wipe skin with spirit or alcohol if you have it.
- Cut boldly through the skin to let out the pus. Cut through the lowest point (when the animal is standing) in the swelling to help drainage.

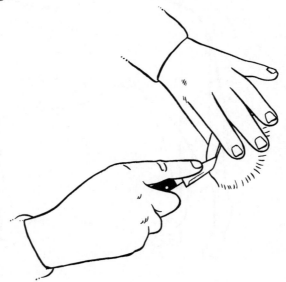

- Make one long, vertical cut. Push a clean finger into the hole to break down tissue and to help release the pus.
- Alternatively, make two cuts in a cross shape so that the skin does not heal up too fast. The aim is for all the infection to drain before the skin heals together.

- Be very careful where you cut around the neck or udder (breast tissue of mare), because there are big veins near the skin in these places that must not be cut.
- Where the pus is spilt dig a hole and bury it.
- Flush the abscess by squirting a dilute solution of iodine into the hole with a syringe. Alternatively, use hydrogen peroxide solution (diluted in water). Oxygen bubbles form and help flush out the infection.
- Continue to bathe the area with hot, salt water several times a day.

If the animal is eating well and is bright after draining the abscess, an antibiotic injection is unnecessary. If the animal is sick give antibiotics as described in the section *Infected wounds*.

8.3   Oedema from allergic reaction

Oedema swellings may be due to allergy, for example, to something eaten or to insect bites. The typical thing about oedema is that it 'pits under pressure'.

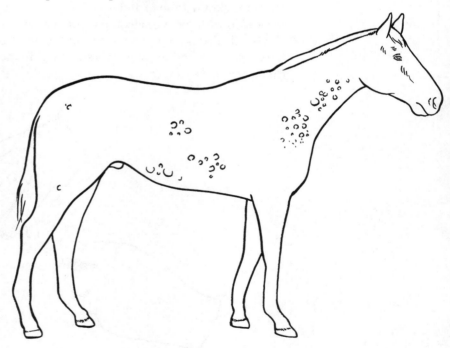

What oedema swellings look like
- These swellings are identified because they pit under pressure. Pressing with a finger or thumb leaves an indentation that stays for some time.
- Oedema swellings are not hot.
- They are not painful.

- They usually develop rapidly, in minutes or hours.
- Horses can develop swellings as wide as large plates.
- Unlike an abscess, there are usually several swellings at the same time.

How to prevent oedema swellings

If you noticed that the horse developed the swellings after eating a particular kind of feed, avoid giving that animal the same thing to eat in future. Allergic swellings are not infectious, and the same food may be perfectly safe for other animals in the group.

How to treat oedema

- Usually no treatment is necessary. It can help to hold a cloth or cotton wool soaked in ice-cold water on the swelling.
- If the animal is distressed, inject a corticosteroid medicine. See the list of medicines at the back of the book.

8.4 Bee stings

Bee stings can cause swellings under the skin. To treat, dissolve sodium bicarbonate in water. Soak cotton wool or a cloth in this and apply to the stung places.

8.5 Haematoma, blood blister

These swellings usually occur after the skin has been banged, resulting in bleeding under the skin.

What haematoma swellings look like

- They are found on the part of the body that has been banged, such as the hip, shoulder or head.
- The swelling is soft at first, but does not 'pit under pressure' like oedema.
- Less painful than an abscess.
- If an empty syringe and needle is put into the lump, blood or serum with blood clots is sucked back.

How to treat a haematoma

An uninfected haematoma swelling can be left alone. As it heals, a haematoma eventually becomes hard. The blood clots and then the serum is absorbed. Later, as scar tissue forms, the swelling shrinks.

If a haematoma becomes infected, treat it like an abscess.

A haematoma sometimes develops between the layers of skin in the ear flap. A haematoma between the layers of skin of the ear flap eventually causes 'cauliflower ear'.

8.6 Tumours and cysts

Sarcoids and melanomas are the names of the commonest types of growth seen on the skin. Melanoma swellings are more often seen on grey/white horses than on horses with dark, pigmented skin.

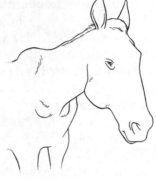

Refer to a veterinarian for treatment. When large melanoma tumours grow in several different parts of the body, euthanasia is appropriate. Other tumours that stick out from the skin are mentioned in the chapter *Diseases and parasites of the skin.*

Cysts contain fluid from a gland. For example, a cyst on the side of the head may contain saliva. Refer to a veterinarian for treatment.

8.7 Hernias and ruptures

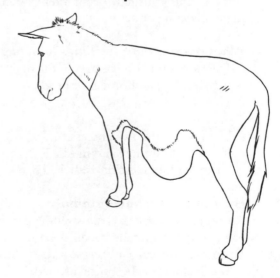

The picture shows a very large hernia or rupture type of swelling in a donkey. Whether large or smaller, the only treatment is surgical. This must be done by a veterinary surgeon. In most cases treatment is not essential, and after some weeks they become painless.

8.8 Purpura

Purpura or purpura haemorrhagica is a rare disease with a variety of signs that include oedema swellings under the skin. It may be mild or very severe. Horses may recover from the mild form in a week, but many cases with the severe form die, in spite of treatment.

What mild purpura looks like
- Oedema swellings under the skin as for allergic reactions,
- stiff muscles,
- horse unwilling to move,
- normal temperature and heart rate.

What severe purpura looks like
- Big oedema swelling, especially over the head and legs.
- The skin may crack over the swelling and ooze liquid.
- Small blood spots under the skin show on the mucous membranes such as the inside of the eyelids (see the section *How to check mucous membranes*).
- Difficult breathing.

What causes purpura
The exact cause is not known. Purpura sometimes follows an infection, particularly strangles.

How to treat purpura
NURSING CARE
Provide comfortable, bedding. Give tasty food (see the section *Thin animals* for advice on feeding). Make sure fresh water is always available. Gentle exercise, for example walking, may help reduce the swellings.

CORTICOSTEROIDS
Corticosteroids should be given until the signs of purpura are reduced.

Inject a corticosteroid drug such as betamethasone or dexamethasone. See list of medicines at the back of the book for doses.

Alternatively, give corticosteroid treatment using prednisolone tablets, crushed and mixed in the food. The dose is 5 mg prednisolone per 10 kg body weight of the animal. Give this dose twice daily.

ANTIBIOTICS
Give injections of penicillin for five days.

9 Diseases and parasites of the skin

9.1 Lice

Adult lice are a few millimetres long, large enough to see moving around between the hairs. Lice bite the skin to feed, which irritates the animal.

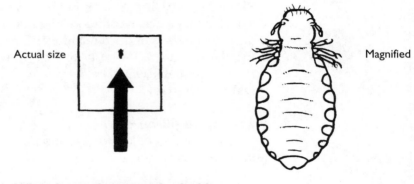

Actual size   Magnified

What lice infestation looks like
- Lice cause itchiness and the animal may rub and lick itself a lot.
- Lice are found especially in the mane and the tail.
- There may be flakes of dead skin in the coat.
- Lice are seen more often on poorly fed and young animals.

One kind of louse (called *Haematopinus*) is larger, about 5 mm long, and these yellow-brown coloured insects can be seen fairly easily. The other kind of louse (called *Damalinia*) is smaller and pale, but can be seen as specks in the hair. With both kinds of louse, their whitish-yellow eggs (nits) can be seen glued on to hairs.

How to prevent lice infestation
- Prevent spread between horses by thoroughly washing all blankets. Saddlery, and other things that contact the animal's skin should be treated with the same drug used to kill lice on the animal. Grooming equipment should be scalded with very hot water.
- Groom the animal regularly. Lice are more common on a thick coat (the winter coat in cool climates) and less often seen after the winter coat is shed. Brush the loose hairs out of the coat. Destroy these hairs (bury or burn) and treat the brush.

How to treat lice infestation

Treatments normally kill the adult lice, but the eggs remain to hatch later. Therefore, give a second treatment two weeks after the first treatment, in order to kill lice which have hatched from the eggs.

- Insecticide sprays or powders (see section at back of book) are effective. See the section *How to spray medicine on to skin* in the chapter *How to give medicines*.
- Ivermectin, more often used against worms, is effective against one type of louse (*Haematopinus*) found on horses, but less effective against the other type.

9.2 Flies

Horses hate flies. Flies irritate them and cause diseases. Flies also carry diseases and spread worms that infect wounds and eyes. The table shows some of the problems caused by flies.

Diseases caused and carried by various types of fly

Diseases caused by the fly	Diseases carried by fly	Type of fly	Actual size	Magnified
Maggots in wounds	Summer sores, habronemiasis	*Calliphora*, etc. blowfly, bluebottle		
Screw worm		*Chrysomya*, *Cochliomyia* screw worm flies		
Sweet itch, irritation	African horse sickness, onchocerciasis	*Culicoides* midge, no-see-um		
Stomach bots, gadding (panic)		*Gasterophilus* bot fly		
Irritation		*Haematopota* cleg		

Diseases caused by the fly	Diseases carried by fly	Type of fly	Actual size	Magnified
Warbles, gadding (panic)		*Hypoderma* gadfly, warble fly		
Irritation	Equine encephalitis	mosquito		
	Habronemiasis (summer sores), eye-worm (*Thelaziasis*)	*Musca* housefly		
Irritation	Onchocerciasis	*Simulium* blackfly		
Irritation	Surra, habronemiasis (summer sores)	*Stomoxys* stable fly		
Irritation from painful bites	Anthrax, equine infectious anaemia, surra	*Tabanus* horsefly		
Irritation	Trypanosomiasis	tsetse fly		
Stings		Wasps, bees, scorpions and centipedes		

How to control flies

- Many flies breed in animal dung. Make dung into compost or burn it. Alternatively spread out the dung so it dries.
- After drying dung in the sun, it can be burned near the animals. The smoke repels flies.
- Where *Stomoxys* flies are a problem, cover or remove rotting vegetation or compost as this type of fly breeds in it.
- Ducks and chickens eat insects. Keeping poultry helps control flies.
- Keep animals away from swampy places in the wet season. Cover water tanks where mosquitoes breed. Keep fish in paddy fields, because fish eat fly larvae.
- Make a back rubber from a sack containing insecticide dust or soaked in insecticide oil. Tie the sack around a tree or post. The animals learn to rub against it. Replace it after about a month.
- Insecticides and chemical insect repellents are effective, but usually too expensive to use routinely. A repellent can be made from kerosene and water (see the section *How to care for a fresh wound*).

Insecticides and fly repellents made from local plants

In many parts of the world, there are plants that contain substances that repel flies. Try to find local knowledge about this. Some examples are:

- Neem tree (*Azadirachta indica*). Neem oil is effective as a repellent and for treating wounds with maggots.
  To make neem oil, remove the outside cover of the seeds. Grind the seeds to make a sticky, brown powder.
  Add a little water and then press and squeeze the paste so that the oil comes out.
- A fly repellent can be made simply by boiling neem leaves and allowing the liquid to cool. Apply to the skin with a cloth.
- Sugar apple tree (*Annona squamosa*). The sugar apple tree is grown in the tropics for its fruit. Take the seeds from the fruit and crush the seeds to make a paste. This paste can be used to kill lice or maggots in a wound.
- Sweet flag plant (*Acorus calamus*). This is a water plant that has sword-shaped leaves and yellow-green flowers in bunches. The thick root stock contains an insecticide. The roots are dried and crushed to powder. The powder can be used to kill lice on animals.

9.3 Mange

Mange is caused by mites, which are very small creatures, only just big enough to see.

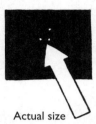

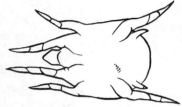

Actual size

Appearance of one kind of mite
seen with a microscope

They burrow into the skin and cause intense irritation, resulting in biting and rubbing by the animal. Mange is less common and severe in horses and donkeys than in some other species, such as goats or camels. Leg mange is the commonest type in horses.

What mange looks like

First type (leg mange, chorioptic mange):

- The skin under the long hair around the heels is affected,
- thickened skin with grey scabs and surface flakes,
- stamping the feet.

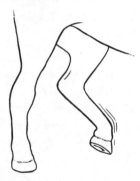

Second type (body mange, psoroptic mange):

- Severe irritation,
- oozing, amber scabs, thickened skin and surface flakes.
- Different types of mange mites prefer different parts of the body, for example:
  - near the long hair at the base of the tail or sides of the mane, or
  - inside the ears.
- Shaking the head if the ears are affected (ticks can also cause this, see the section *Ticks*),
- rubbing of mane or tail,
- eventually, affected skin may have thick scabs heaped up beneath the hair.

Third type (scab mites, sarcoptic mange):
- Crusty, grey-brown hairless patches,
- severe irritation resulting in biting and rubbing,
- areas affected vary, but it usually occurs on parts of the body with short hair, such as the head and neck.

To be sure an animal has mange, it is necessary to see the mites by using a microscope to examine a scraping of the skin. See the section *How to collect samples for laboratory tests.*

How to prevent mange
Mange is passed from one horse to another by contact between them, or by using the same grooming equipment or tack. Therefore, treat infected cases and keep them separate from other animals until cured. Do not use the same grooming equipment on other animals. Treat grooming equipment with insecticide.

How to treat mange
Sprays used for ticks work against mange, especially the mange mite type (psoroptic mange). See the list of suitable chemicals at the back of the book. Apply once per week and give at least four treatments. Mix the chemical carefully according to the instructions. Wear rubber gloves or plastic bags over your hands. Use a cloth to rub the mixture into the affected areas or use a sprayer. See the section *How to spray medicine on to skin* in the chapter *How to give medicines.*

Ivermectin is effective against the scab mite type (sarcoptic mange). It may also cure the other types.

9.4 Harvest mites, heel bug

Harvest mites are similar in size to mange and scab mites, but harvest mites live in the grass. The young stages of these creatures feed on animals' skin. They get on to the legs or face when the animals graze.

What infestation looks like
- Intense irritation.
- Small, red-orange clusters of mites may be seen on the face or lower legs.
- The skin may ooze and drip.
- The heel is often affected.
- It occurs in summer in places with a cold winter.

How to prevent infestation
With a solution used for ticks, wash the lower legs and face two or three times a week in the season. Replace the bedding if it is straw or hay that may have forage mites in it.

How to treat infestation

In countries with a cold climate, the disease disappears in the cold season when the mites are no longer in the grass. Spraying or washing with a chemical for killing ticks (see list at the back of the book) can give instant relief. See the section *How to spray medicine on to skin* in the chapter *How to give medicines*.

9.5 Sweet itch

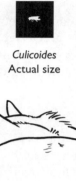

Culicoides
Actual size

This condition is an allergic reaction to bites of midges or gnats (*Culicoides*).

Sensitive horses rub their manes and tails because of severe irritation.

What sweet itch looks like

- Usually only one horse in a group is affected.
- The skin is pink, inflamed and in thick folds.
- The mane, back and tail are affected.
- The tail may be rubbed raw.
- The tail base may look like an old scrubbing brush.

How to prevent sweet itch

- The biting insects that cause sweet itch feed in the late afternoon and at night. Therefore, from mid-afternoon, put the horse inside under a roof. This will greatly reduce midge attack.
- Insect netting over the windows will keep midges out, but only if the holes in the netting are small enough. Midges can get through mosquito netting.
- Insect repellents or insecticide, such as synthetic pyrethroids, can be applied to the mane, back and tail.

There is no cure. Affected horses will always have this problem when bitten by midges. In cold climates, the disease gets better in the winter when flies are not around.

9.6 Pinworm

This disease affects stabled horses. A gut worm (*Oxyuris equi*) causes it. The female worm is up to 15 mm long and crawls out of the anus and lays its eggs under the tail. Large numbers of eggs are sometimes seen under the tail and are known as 'rust'.

What pinworm infestation looks like

- Severe irritation under the tail.
- The horse rubs its tail against posts or trees.

How to treat pinworm infestation

- Wash around the anus with soap or mild disinfectant solution.
- Treat the horse with a medicine against worms (see list at the back of the book), for example:
  - piperazine citrate, dose 200 mg per kg body weight,
  - ivermectin,
  - fenbendazole (Panacur).

9.7 Ticks

Ticks attach to the skin and feed on blood. Ticks spend more time in the pasture, off the animal, than feeding on it.

Diseases caused by ticks

- Usually they do not cause much damage, but they can carry diseases, such as babesiosis.
- The bites can become infected, resulting in an abscess.
- Sometimes ticks get into the ears and cause head-shaking and distress.
- Rarely, some ticks cause paralysis. This has been seen in foals in Australia.

How to treat ticks

PICK OFF BY HAND

Remove from the animal by hand picking. Do this carefully so that tick mouth-parts are not left in the skin.

USE CHEMICALS TO KILL THE TICKS

Ticks can be killed with chemicals that are more commonly used on cattle (see list at the back of the book). Some of these chemicals are dangerous to animals and people, so follow instructions carefully.

- The chemicals can be applied with a sprayer. See the section *How to spray medicine on to skin* in the chapter *How to give medicines*.
- Chemicals to kill ticks are also sold as 'pour-on' oils. These are easy to use, but may not have been tested on horses.
- Chemical can be applied using a sponge or cloth. Mix the chemical in a bucket using the amount recommended for dipping or spraying. Wear rubber gloves or plastic bags over your hands.
- Ear ticks can be treated with tick chemical sold for dips or sprays, but mixed with oil instead of water. Use the same dilution instructed by the manufacturer when mixing with water, but mix with vegetable cooking oil. Squirt a few millilitres directly into the ear using a syringe without a needle.

9.8 Warts

Warts most commonly occur in young animals on the lips, nostrils, eyelids, legs or genitals. Normally no treatment is necessary and they disappear after a few months.

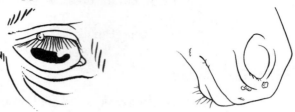

If they are a problem, for example, by interfering with the harness, tie cotton thread tightly around the base. This cuts off the blood supply and the wart drops off after a few days. Be sure the horse is vaccinated against tetanus before doing this.

9.9 Sarcoids

What sarcoids look like
- Lumps that first appear as hard bumps under the skin.
- They grow to about 3 cm diameter, sometimes bigger.
- As they get bigger the skin on the surface becomes raw.

Call vet!

How to treat sarcoids
A trained veterinarian, who may use surgery or a cell-killing cream, should treat sarcoids.

9.10 Warbles

Warbles are bumps containing the larvae of the warble fly (*Hypoderma*). These flies live in the northern hemisphere and mainly parasitize cattle. See the section *Flies* for a picture of a warble fly.

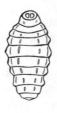

Warble fly larva
Actual size

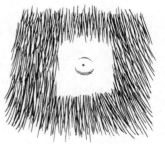

Bump or warble
Half actual size

What warbles look like

- Bumps, called warbles, 1 or 2 cm wide under the skin on the back.
- There is a small hole in the centre of the bump through which the maggot breathes.
- The bumps appear in the spring.
- Warbles are painful and may prevent work.

How to treat warbles

With a sharp knife, such as a razor blade, make the breathing hole larger. Gently squeeze the bump and remove the larva using tweezers. Be *very* careful not to break the larva.

9.11 Other growths, tumours

Tumours or cancerous growths are incurable. They grow progressively. Tumours occur in older horses.

What tumours look like

Melanoma, the most common kind of tumour:
- usually affects white/grey horses,
- black or brown lumps appear under the skin,
- these lumps may start under the tail, but later grow in other sites.

Other types of tumour:
- can also cause lumps under the skin, or
- can cause pinkish growths in animals with pink skin, for example, around the eyes.

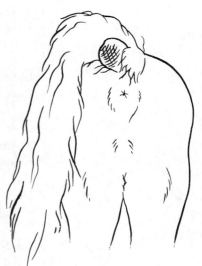

How to treat tumours

Call vet!

- Surgery by a veterinarian is the only treatment. If it only affects one place, surgery may prevent it from spreading more.
- If melanoma growths have become large and have spread to involve several places on the body, euthanasia is recommended.

9.12 Ringworm, dermatomycosis

This disease usually self-cures after around three months. It is very infectious and some forms can infect people. It is not caused by a worm, but by a fungus. It tends to grow out in circular rings, hence the name.

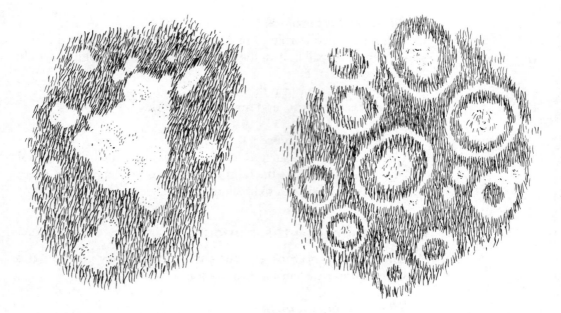

What ringworm looks like
* First, round areas of raised skin appear.
* Next, the hair mats together.
* After about a week the hair falls out leaving a roughly circular patch of grey skin.
* There is some irritation, but not severe in most animals.
* It usually starts on the belly and can spread to the neck, head or rump.

How to prevent ringworm
* Do not let healthy animals rub against animals with ringworm.
* Do not share the blankets or saddles of animals with ringworm. Do not groom all animals with the same equipment. Wash your hands with soap after touching an infected horse. (It is better to wear rubber gloves when grooming a horse with ringworm so that you are less likely to catch it yourself.)
* Clean their housing and posts that they rub against with 'Clorox' bleach (sodium hypochlorite solution).

How to treat ringworm
* Most cases recover naturally, after a long period, so treatment is not always necessary.
* Severe cases can be treated with griseofulvin (Fulcin) added to the feed, but do not feed to pregnant mares.
* Treat affected skin with a disinfectant solution, for example, chlorhexidine solution (25 ml in 1 litre of water) or sodium hypochlorite solution (100 ml in 1 litre of water). Put the solution on to the ringworm with a sponge or cloth.

9.13 Sunburn, photosensitization

Badly sunburnt skin can occur after eating plants containing substances that make skin sensitive to sunlight. It can also be the result of liver disease, which can in turn follow poisoning with certain plants, such as *Senecio* species, like ragwort. It affects horses that have patches of white hair or pink skin.

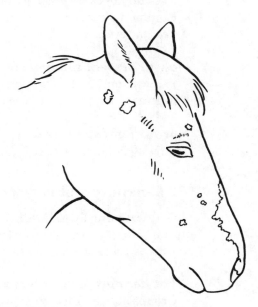

What photosensitization looks like
- Reddening of skin that does not have dark pigment, that is, where the hair is white and on pink skin of the eyelids, ears and lips.
- The skin becomes thickened and scabby.
- The surface layer flakes off.

How to prevent photosensitization
Keep susceptible animals in the shade during daylight. Avoid access to areas known to have plants that cause this problem, such as *Senecio* species or wild clovers.

How to treat photosensitization
If poisonous plants have badly damaged the liver, there is no effective treatment. See the section *Liver disease*.

9.14 Summer sores, habronemiasis, bursatti

The young forms of certain stomach worms of horses cause summer sores when they get into wounds. Flies, such as the housefly or stable fly, carry the larvae to the wound. The disease is sometimes known as swamp cancer or bursatti. The same worms cause swellings and raw ulcers on the face, below the eyes (see the chapter *Eye problems*).

What summer sores looks like

- Lumps that grow up to 25 cm diameter and have a sunken centre.
- The lumps look like proud flesh covered with a thin, greyish skin.
- They do not cause much irritation.
- Common places where the lumps grow are under the belly and near the eyes.

How to prevent summer sores

- Remove dung and rotting vegetation where flies breed.
- Keep all wounds clean. Infected wounds are more attractive to flies.

How to treat summer sores

Treat with ivermectin, dose 0.2 mg per kg body weight.

9.15 Dermatophilosis, streptothricosis

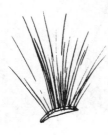

This disease usually follows heavy wetting of the skin, which helps the infection to start in the surface layers of the skin. It is sometimes known as 'rain scald' or 'mud fever'.

What dermatophilosis looks like

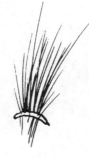

- Groups of hairs are matted together in a tuft, like a small paint brush.
- Tufts usually appear first on the legs or belly but can be on other parts of the body.
- If the tuft of hair is pulled off the hairs are stuck together by a scab.
- Where a matted tuft of hair was removed the skin is moist, pink and may bleed.
- In older, healing dermatophilosis, the hairs grow with the scab around them.

How to prevent dermatophilosis

Keep the animals dry. Do not allow them to stand in mud.

How to treat dermatophilosis

- Many animals recover without treatment, particularly when kept dry.
- Recovery is more rapid if the scabs are soaked in povidone-iodine solution and removed by hand. This may be painful, and, unless the animal is very quiet, restrain with a twitch (see the section *How to restrain horses and donkeys*). After removing scabs, apply antibiotic ointment.
- Intramuscular injections of penicillin, for five days.

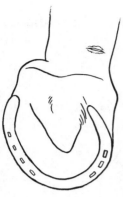

9.16 Cracked heel

This condition occurs just above the heel. The cracks may become deep and infected and the horse may become lame. It may be a form of dermatophilosis.

How to prevent cracked heel

It occurs when a horse has been standing in wet mud or when the horse's legs have been washed frequently and not dried. If the animal is on wet land, put some petroleum jelly (Vaseline) on the skin every few days. This is not necessary if the weather is dry and if the heels do not get wet where the animal walks and stands.

Cracked heel may also occur when an animal has not been properly hobbled (tied by its lower legs). Make sure that rope used for this is dry and soft.

How to treat cracked heel

- Wash with warm water and soap to remove the scabs. Dry the area well with clean cloths.
- Put on some petroleum jelly or zinc oxide ointment. Repeat every few days.
- If lame, rest the horse. Even if not lame, do not work the animal hard until its heel cracks have healed completely.
- Remove ropes from the lower legs until cracks have healed.

9.17 Vesicular stomatitis

Donkeys and horses can get vesicular stomatitis, which causes blisters in and around the mouth. It occurs in North, Central and South America, usually in late summer. The disease is transmitted by flies.

What vesicular stomatitis looks like

- Dribbling.
- The animal is not willing to eat.
- Blisters appear on the gums, tongue and lips.
- Blisters may also appear above the hooves or on the teats.
- Recovery occurs after about a week.

How to prevent vesicular stomatitis

- Keep animals in stables with mosquito netting.
- Keep uninfected animals away from any with the disease.

How to treat vesicular stomatitis

There is no direct treatment. Nursing care is needed: provide the animal with soft food and keep it comfortable until it recovers.

9.18 Fly-blown wounds and screw worm

See the section *Fly-blown wounds, screw worm* in the chapter *How to treat wounds.*

9.19 Fistulous withers and poll evil

These conditions are names of a deep infection on the top of the head or in the neck (withers).

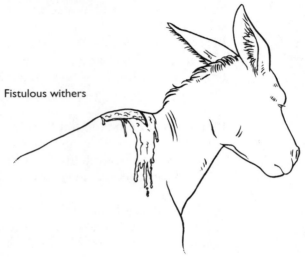

Fistulous withers

What fistulous withers and poll evil look like

A creamy, pus discharge bursts out through the skin. It is seen at the top of the neck from the poll infection or in front of and above the shoulders. ('Poll' is a name for the top of the head. 'Withers' is a name for the top of the neck above the shoulders.)

How to prevent fistulous withers and poll evil

- The infections follow injury.
- Fistulous withers is most commonly caused by badly fitting harness. See the section *Pack animals*. Make sure a pack saddle is applied so that it does not move forward and cause injury to the withers.
- Poll evil can follow banging the head on the top of a door frame. Avoid these injuries with good door design.
- Wash your hands thoroughly with soap after touching these lesions and before touching other animals.

How to treat fistulous withers and poll evil

Call vet!

These conditions are difficult to treat and require radical surgery by a veterinarian, as well as antibiotics. The deep cutting out of infected tissue must be done by a veterinary surgeon.

9.20 Epizootic lymphangitis (pseudoglanders)

This disease is found chiefly in Asia and northern Africa. It affects horses and mules especially when kept crowded together. Donkeys rarely get it.

The infection gets into the body through damage to the skin and can be carried by biting flies.

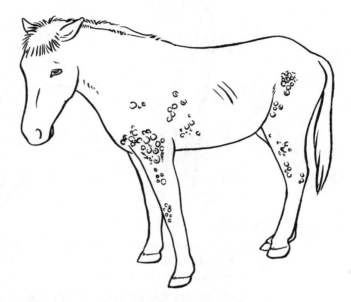

What epizootic lymphangitis looks like

- Painful lumps develop under the skin, especially on the legs, but also on the head, neck and shoulders, usually where the tack or harness contacts the skin.
- After some weeks, the lumps burst and yellow pus drips from them.
- Lumps may appear on the nostrils, but not up inside the nose (as in glanders).
- Between the lumps there are thickened tubes (lymph vessels) under the skin.
- The animal becomes thin and loses condition.

The disease lasts for several months to a year. Animals can recover without treatment, but about 10% of cases die.

How to prevent epizootic lymphangitis

- Keep affected animals as far away from others as possible.
- Euthanase severe cases to reduce the source of infection to others.
- Disinfect harnesses and all equipment for grooming, as for glanders.
- Control insects (see the section *Flies*).

Treatment
There is no effective treatment. Clean abscesses with iodine solution.

9.21   Ulcerative lymphangitis

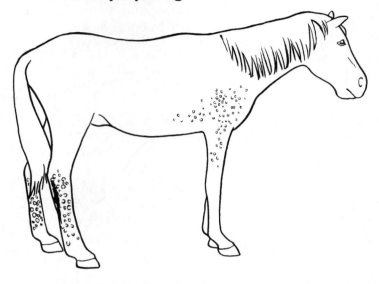

This disease occurs in Africa, North and South America, the Middle East and the Indian subcontinent. It mainly affects horses, but can affect donkeys and mules too. The infection starts in skin wounds and is more common when animals have been standing in muddy places.

What ulcerative lymphangitis looks like
- Swollen legs with bumps that may be in rows.
- The bumps burst and creamy pus comes out of them.
- The hind legs below the hocks are most commonly affected.

How to prevent ulcerative lymphangitis
- Keep infected animals away from other ones.
- Disinfect all equipment that comes into contact with the animals as for glanders.
- If possible, do not keep animals in muddy places for long periods.
- Control insects (see the section *Flies*).

How to treat ulcerative lymphangitis
- Wash out the sores and lumps with iodine solution or povidone-iodine solution.
- Give antibiotic injections, for example, penicillin or sulphonamides.

Severe cases do not always recover.

9.22 Glanders

This disease is rare, but occurs occasionally in the Middle East and parts of Asia. Glanders affects the skin and the lungs. Donkeys and mules may die within two weeks, but horses are less likely to die from glanders. People can also catch glanders, but human infection is rare.

What glanders looks like
Sometimes it affects the lungs more, sometimes the skin. Some or all of the following signs are seen:

- fever,
- coughing and difficulty breathing,
- discharge from the nose, watery at first and later thicker with blood tinges,
- lumps, 1 cm wide, appear in the nostrils and break open,
- when the lumps heal, there is a star-shaped scar inside the nose,
- lumps, 1–2 cm wide, on the skin of the legs or belly,
- thickened tubes (lymph vessels), which run between the lumps, can be felt under the skin,
- these lumps also burst open and release a sticky, honey-like discharge,
- affected legs become swollen and painful.

If a horse that had glanders is looked at post-mortem, 1 cm wide balls can be seen in its lungs. These balls are either red or yellow inside.

How to prevent glanders
- Destroy affected animals and bury their bodies.
- Disinfect the stables and any buckets, grooming equipment or tack that has been contaminated with discharges from the glanders lumps. Burn any dry bedding.
- Vets may test in-contact animals (mallein test) to detect any with early infections. These cases are destroyed to prevent glanders from occurring in the group.

How to treat glanders
Inject sulphadiazine daily for 20 days.

Do not treat if the aim is to prevent other animals from getting glanders because, when they recover after treatment, they may remain as a source of infection.

9.23 Pythiosis, Florida horse leeches

This disease is found in places with a hot climate, usually humid, coastal areas. These places include parts of South America, the USA and Australia. A fungus of plants that gets into a wound and spreads there causes pythiosis.

What pythiosis looks like
- A wound that quickly becomes much worse and larger,
- very itchy,
- thick, bloody liquid drips out and hangs from the wound in strings.

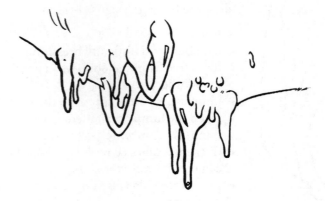

How to treat pythiosis
It is difficult to treat and not all cases recover.

- Apply iodine solution or povidone-iodine to the affected area twice daily for at least a month.
- A veterinarian should surgically remove the infected tissue.

10 Diseases affecting breathing

10.1 Flu (equine influenza, stable cough)

Flu, which is caused by viruses, leads to a severe cough. It sometimes spreads through populations of horses and donkeys as an epidemic.

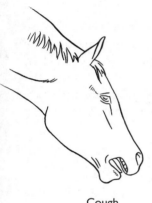

Cough

What flu looks like
- Usually more than one animal is affected.
- First, the animal has a raised temperature for a few days. At this time, there are no special signs, but the animal is a bit less alert and less willing to work.
- Then, a cough begins. The horse coughs frequently as though its throat tickles.
- There is a watery discharge from the nostrils. After a few days this becomes thicker and yellowish.
- Now the cough becomes more severe. It is a dry, hacking cough that lasts for two or three weeks.

How flu spreads
- Infected horses cough out virus particles. Other horses close by breathe the coughed air and easily catch the infection.
- People who handle the sick animals also take the infection to other horses.

How to prevent flu
Vaccines are available against this disease. One injection is given to start vaccination, followed by a second injection six weeks later. Protection lasts for a year. Booster injections can be given every 12–15 months to keep up the protection. Sometimes tetanus vaccine is combined in the same injection.

If the cough has started in a group of horses, do not let uninfected horses come near sick ones until they are better. Anybody who is looking after sick horses should not handle other ones.

At the end of the infection in a group of horses, carefully clean all equipment (including all harnesses, water buckets and food containers, etc.) and leave them in the sun to dry. Any buildings where the horses were tied should be cleaned out and disinfected so that the source of infection does not remain.

How to treat flu

- Rest the animal. Do not work it while it has a cough or for a week after. If you do, its full recovery will be delayed and it may never fully get better.
- Feed soft food that is easily swallowed, for example, bran soaked in water. Tempt the animal to eat with food you know it likes.
- House sick animals in a dry, comfortable place without a cold draught.
- Put a rug or blanket on the horse if the weather is cool.
- Antibiotics are not normally necessary. Injections of penicillin with streptomycin can be given. Do treat with antibiotics if the animal is still coughing after three weeks.

As with the common cold that people catch, there is no effective treatment for this kind of virus infection. The animal needs to be kept comfortable and nursed through the infection until it gets better.

In more serious cases antibiotic injections are given so that the virus infection is not made worse by secondary infections with bacteria. Unlike virus infections, bacterial infections can be treated with antibiotics.

10.2 Viral nose infections

There are some infections that mainly affect the passages through the nose. Infection here causes liquid to run from the nose without much coughing.

Three names for these infections are rhinitis, rhinopneumonitis and equine herpes virus abortion. All three are caused by infectious particles called viruses. The rhinitis virus only infects inside the nose. The herpes virus can also infect a foal developing inside its mother and can cause an abortion.

What these nose infections look like

When the infection starts:
- fever (up to 41°C for a horse),
- the animal behaves in a dull and depressed way,
- discharge from the nose is watery at first and then thicker and yellow-white,
- sometimes the legs become very swollen during infection.

From one month after the first infection was seen:
- foals may be born which are not fully formed,
- usually these foals are born dead, but sometimes they survive for a few hours.

How to prevent these nose infections

- Keep any animals with a discharge from the nose or a cough separate from others, especially from pregnant mares.

- A vaccine is available, but is not always effective.

How to treat these nose infections
- Rest and nursing, as for flu (above). Horses should be rested for at least one month.
- Antibiotic injections, such as penicillin with streptomycin, should be given against secondary infections.

10.3 Strangles

At first this disease looks like flu, but the cough disappears after one or two days and then pus comes from the nostrils and the lymph glands behind the jaw swell.

What strangles looks like
At first, the horse has:
- a high temperature,
- a watery discharge from the nose and
- a cough.

After one or two days:
- the cough disappears,
- swallowing is difficult (because of a sore throat),
- thick, creamy, white pus drips from both nostrils.

Then:
- lymph nodes around the neck swell, and
- they become hot and very painful,
- after getting bigger for a few days they form abscesses (see the section *Abscess and how to recognize and treat it*).

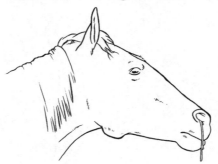

About two weeks after the start of the infection:
- these abscesses burst and creamy white pus (the same as is seen coming out of the nose) drips down the skin,
- the animal becomes brighter and recovers when the pus starts to come out from the abscesses,
- occasionally, at this stage the animal gets a reaction to the infection (see the section *Purpura*).

How to prevent strangles

If one horse in a group has strangles, it is very difficult to stop it from spreading to others. However, these measures will help prevent other animals from catching it:

- If the disease has broken out, take healthy horses away from infected ones. The pus that comes out of the nose or abscesses carries the infection. Make sure you wash it carefully off your hands and clothes before going near another horse.
- Every day, scrub all equipment (harnesses, buckets, brushes) with disinfectant and put it in the sun to dry. Remove all bedding on to which pus may have dripped and burn it.
- Take the temperatures of all horses nearby twice every day. If you find an animal with a raised temperature, treat it daily with antibiotic (penicillin injection) for three to five days to prevent the disease.

How to treat strangles

- Rest.
- Nursing as for flu above. Remember the infection causes a sore throat and so the animal should be offered soft, moist food.
- 'Steaming' helps make the discharge less thick. Do this by pouring boiling water (you can add a few drops of eucalyptus oil) on to some hay in the bottom of a feed bag. It is best to use an old feed bag with holes which allow air in. Hold the top of the bag around the horse's head so it breathes in more steam. The animal might panic, so stand with it while the steam bag is on.

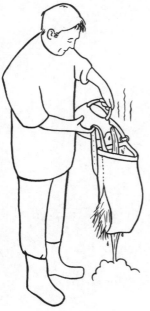
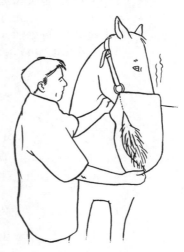

- Antibiotics must be used carefully, if at all. Do not use antibiotics before the infected nodes have burst and pus is seen dripping down the skin. If you inject antibiotic early, it may just partly clear the infection in these abscesses. The infection might then linger for much longer and come out later in several places.

10.4 Sinusitis

The 'sinuses' are hollow spaces inside bones of the skull. Sometimes infection occurs inside these spaces. This is sinusitis.

The position of hollow sinuses in the bones of a horse's head is shown in the picture.

What sinusitis looks like

Thick mucus, dripping from one or both nostrils is the main sign of sinusitis.

What causes sinusitis

- The animal has usually had an infection like strangles or flu and then not completely recovered.
- Sinusitis can be associated with a cheek tooth from the top row that has become infected or has not grown down properly. If this happens there will normally be a runny nose only on one side, which is the side with the problem tooth.

How to prevent sinusitis

If an animal has strangles or flu, give proper nursing care and enough rest. Then sinusitis is less likely to follow.

How to treat sinusitis

When a lot of infected pus and mucus has developed inside a sinus, it is difficult for antibiotics given by injection to reach the infection. It is necessary to try to clear the pus and mucus from the sinus, so the treatment should include steaming or trephining, as well as antibiotics.

Call vet!

- When the horse keeps its head down, the sinuses drain better. Therefore, put the animal's feed on the ground or put it out to graze.
- Steaming is described in the treatment of strangles. It will help make the discharge less thick and help it to drain out of the sinuses.
- Antibiotic injections. Because it is difficult to get the antibiotic to where the infection is, it is usually necessary to give a long course of injections, for example, daily for two weeks. Use broad-spectrum antibiotic such as penicillin with streptomycin.
- It is important to rest the animal and keep it in a comfortable place until it has recovered. Turn it out to graze.
- Trephining, which only a veterinarian can do. It involves drilling a hole through the side of the head, usually just below the eye, so that the sinuses can be washed out with an appropriate solution.
- Remove the problem cheek tooth. (This is also a job that can only be done by a veterinarian with expertise in equine dentistry. The technique requires a general anaesthetic and removal of the tooth through a flap opened in the bone on the side of the face.)

10.5 Lung worms

Worms in the breathing tubes can cause coughing that lasts for several months. Lung worms often infect donkeys, but donkeys, unlike horses, often do not become ill.

What lung worm disease looks like

- Coughing, sometimes quite violent.
- The disease can go on for months.
- After each bout of coughing, the lips are wet with saliva.
- In countries with a cold winter, the disease occurs in the summer or autumn and most horses recover by winter.
- Treatment and recovery after giving worm medicine confirms that lung worm was the cause of coughing.

How to prevent lung worm

- Where lung worm is a problem, avoid keeping horses with donkeys.
- If horses are kept with donkeys, treat the donkeys for worms. In places where there is a cold winter, do this in the spring just

before the ground warms up, because, in warmer conditions, the infective larvae develop on the grass and infect other animals.
- Treat animals regularly for worms.

How to treat lung worm
Use a drug for deworming, for example:

- ivermectin, dose 0.2 mg (200 µg) per kg body weight, or
- fenbendazole (Panacur), dose 15 mg per kg body weight, or
- thiabendazole (Thibenzole), dose 440 mg per kg body weight and repeat after two days.

10.6 Chronic pulmonary disease (CPD), broken wind, heaves

This disease is also called COPD or chronic obstructive pulmonary disease. It occurs where horses are housed and fed hay. The disease does not spread from horse to horse. It is caused by an allergy to mould or dust. This disease may develop after an infection such as flu.

What CPD looks like
- The horse is kept in a house with dry hay or straw around.
- It is bright and well in itself and has a normal temperature.
- Its breathing is faster than normal (often more than 20 breaths per minute for an adult horse).
- The horse makes more effort than normal to breathe out.
- Occasionally there is mild coughing (so the disease can look like lung worm disease) especially when the horse starts to trot.
- The disease can continue for months.
- There may be a discharge from the nose.

How to prevent CPD
Most horses will never get this disease, which is an allergic reaction to dry, dusty hay that affects some individual animals. For an individual that does get CPD, follow the advice on treatment, below.

How to treat CPD
- Prevent access to dusty hay.
- Keep the horse outside under shelter, but not in a closed box.
- Before taking it to the horse, soak hay in water by putting a net of hay in a tank or large bucket.
- Feed something else if possible, but, if hay is given, only feed the best, new hay.
- Store hay away from where the horse lives.
- Do not use straw for bedding. Use wood sawdust or shredded newspaper or earth.

Other important infections

11.1 Tetanus or 'lock-jaw'

Tetanus follows infection of a wound. The wound may have been small, such as a puncture wound from a nail, and may not have been noticed. Signs of tetanus may not be seen until some weeks after the wound. Tetanus causes muscle contractions (stiffness) and often results in death.

What tetanus looks like

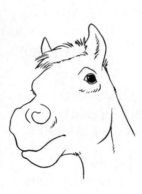

- The horse has a frightened expression.
- Eyes are slit-like, the third eyelid stays partly across the eye (it is normally only just visible at the inside corner of the eye).
- The pupils, the black part in the centre of the eye, stay wide open in bright light.
- The ears stick up and are stiff.
- As tetanus develops, the horse becomes stiffer. It stands with its legs spread out.

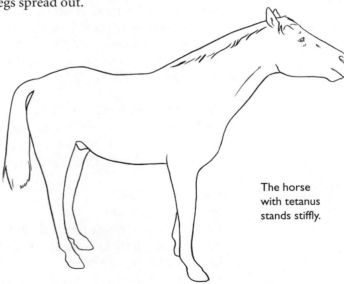

The horse with tetanus stands stiffly.

- The jaw cannot open, it cannot chew and strands of saliva may hang from the mouth.
- Quivering contractions of its muscles happen after stimulation, such as sudden noise or bright light.

- The temperature is usually normal.
- The horse stands for as long as it can. When it collapses with exhaustion, it soon dies. Most cases die in three to ten days. Donkeys have better survival rates than horses.

How to prevent tetanus

Tetanus is prevented by vaccination with tetanus toxoid. Two injections three to four weeks apart are normally required to protect an adult horse. For vaccinating foals, follow the manufacturer's instructions.

Immunity may be long, although vaccine manufacturers may recommend boosting the vaccination every two years. Vaccination even once in an animal's life greatly reduces the risk of it ever getting tetanus.

If an unvaccinated horse has a wound, temporary prevention can be provided by an injection of tetanus antitoxin.

How to treat tetanus

Treatment is rarely successful in horses. Many donkeys and some horses recover if kept quiet and given good nursing care.

- Put the horse in a quiet, dimly lit stable.
- Hand-feed soft, easily swallowed feed, such as bran mash and fresh green leaves.
- Sedate the horse. Give injections of acetylpromazine, up to 0.1 mg/kg body weight every four to six hours according to effect.
- Inject penicillin.
- Give a large dose of tetanus antitoxin.

Prevention, by vaccination, is much more effective than treatment for tetanus.

11.2 Rabies

In most parts of the world rabies is not a common disease of horses or donkeys. It causes unusual behaviour and then, in most cases, death in three to ten days. It is a dangerous disease, and fatal to people who get it.

If you are bitten by a horse you suspect has rabies, or if its saliva contacts even a small wound on your skin, scrub your wound with soap for five minutes *as soon as you can*. Ask a doctor for advice about whether you need more treatment.

How animals get rabies

The disease is caught from the bite of an infected animal, usually a dog. It is sometimes caught from a wild animal such as a fox. In Latin America, it is also spread by vampire bats.

What rabies looks like

The signs do not appear until at least two weeks and up to several months after the bite from the infected animal.

Signs vary. These signs of rabies infection may be seen:

- grinding the teeth and whinnying, or
- a 'dumb' form when the animal stops eating, appears depressed, or
- a 'furious' form when the animal becomes excited and manic, or
- the horse may become paralysed and be unable to stand.

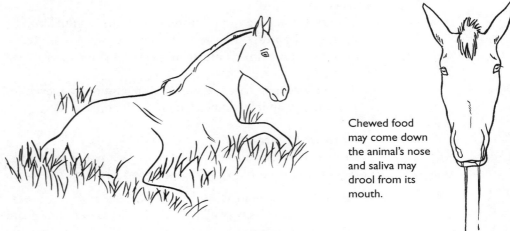

Chewed food may come down the animal's nose and saliva may drool from its mouth.

How to prevent rabies

A vaccine is available, but is normally used only on animals in high-risk areas.

How to treat rabies

Treatment is not effective. Euthanasia is recommended. Take care not to be bitten.

If a horse has been bitten by an animal known or suspected to have rabies, a series of injections of rabies vaccine can stop the disease occuring. After the bite, vaccine is injected on day 0, day 3, day 7, day 14, day 28 and day 30.

11.3 Anthrax

Anthrax is an infection of the blood. Other species, such as cattle, usually die quickly after the signs of anthrax appear. Horses and donkeys may be ill for a long time and do not always die.

What anthrax looks like

- A high temperature (up to 106°F or 41°C) at first.
- A rapid pulse (80–90 for an adult horse) and rapid breathing.
- Colic signs, such as kicking at the belly.
- Large swellings, especially around the neck.

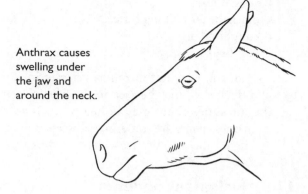

Anthrax causes
swelling under
the jaw and
around the neck.

Laboratory
needed!

- The diagnosis of anthrax is confirmed by using a microscope to examine a blood smear. See the section *How to collect samples for laboratory tests*.

How to prevent anthrax

Anthrax can be prevented by vaccination. In areas where anthrax is common, an injection is given once a year.

The anthrax-causing germ lives for many years in the soil. Animals can get the disease when they eat a bit of contaminated soil with grass. An animal that has died of anthrax can be a source of infection for many years. It is possible to reduce the contamination of the soil with the germs from an animal that has died of anthrax:

- Stop vultures, dogs, etc. from opening the body. Put thorn bushes over the body or guard it for a few days. In hot countries, the germs will die inside the body of the animal in a few days. If the blood of an anthrax case is not allowed to contact the air, the germs in the blood cannot turn into spores, the form that stays on in the soil.
- The alternative is to bury it deeply, about 2 metres deep, and cover it with lime.

How to treat anthrax

Give injections of antibiotics such as penicillin.

11.4 Tuberculosis

There are three types of tuberculosis: the human type, the bovine (cattle) type and the avian (bird) type. Horses do sometimes get the avian or bovine form. However, the disease is not as common in horses and donkeys as in some other species.

What tuberculosis looks like

The signs are not unique to this disease. For example, some of these may be seen:

- weight loss,
- diarrhoea for a long time,
- coughing, or
- stiff neck.

If an animal with tuberculosis is examined post-mortem, abscesses in a thick shell may be seen in the liver, spleen or lymph nodes near the intestine. There may be many small abscesses or one or more large ones. There are sometimes abscesses in the bones or lungs.

There is no effective treatment.

11.5   Malignant oedema

Malignant oedema is a gangrenous infection of wounds that usually results in death.

What malignant oedema looks like
- Swelling of the wound, with gas bubbles.
- Very dull animal, with a rapid pulse.
- Later the animal becomes colder, shivery and dies.

How to prevent malignant oedema
Keep wounds clean. If castrating a horse, perform the operation on clean ground or grass.

How to treat malignant oedema
Treatment is rarely effective, but try giving large doses of penicillin. Wash the wound with antiseptic. See the section *Infected wounds*.

11.6   Babesiosis, piroplasmosis

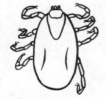

Tick magnified. Some ticks carry babesiosis.

Babesia spp. are microscopic parasites that live inside red blood cells and then destroy them. *Babesia* get into the horse or donkey's body when ticks on its skin are feeding on its blood. The disease is found in many tropical and subtropical parts of the world, including southern Europe, Florida, Latin America, the Caribbean and Asia.

What babesiosis looks like
- Fever,
- the animal is unwilling to move around and stops eating,
- yellow mucous membranes (jaundice),
- small blood spots under the skin of mucous membranes,
- red urine,
- oedema swelling of the face and body.

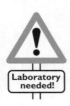

Laboratory needed!

Diagnosis is confirmed in the laboratory by seeing the parasites inside red blood cells (see the section *Blood smear*).

The animal may die just one or two days after the first signs are seen.

Infection without disease

Animals growing up where there are ticks and where the infection is widespread do not normally get ill from the disease. They become infected as foals and acquire a type of immunity.

Animals that never met the disease as foals are at great risk if brought, as an adult, to an area with ticks and babesiosis. Animals that do have some immunity can get the disease if they are stressed, for example, by over-work.

How to prevent babesiosis

There is no vaccine, but making sure foals less than six months old graze with other animals on pasture with ticks should mean that they get infected at an age when they will not get serious disease. Should they get the signs described above, treat them.

How to treat babesiosis

Intramuscular injections of imidocarb (Imizol). See list of *Medicines for treating infections* at the back of the book for the dose.

11.7 Viral encephalomyelitis diseases

Members of a group of similar diseases are each caused by a different virus. These viruses can infect humans too.

Where viral encephalomyelitis diseases occur

Disease name	Where it occurs
Eastern equine encephalomyelitis (EEE)	Eastern USA
Western equine encephalomyelitis (WEE)	Western USA, Canada
Venezuelan equine encephalomyelitis (VEE)	Latin America
Japanese equine encephalomyelitis (JEE)	Asia (from India to the Far East)
West Nile encephalomyelitis (WNE)	Africa, western Asia and southern Europe (e.g. Carmargue)

Viruses living in birds, reptiles or rodents cause these diseases. Infection of horses and donkeys (or humans) can follow a bite from a mosquito that has already fed on one of the wildlife species having the virus.

Mosquitos carry
encephalomyelitis viruses

What viral encephalomyelitis looks like

Some of the following signs are seen:

- fever up to 41°C (106°F),
- stops eating,
- various changed behaviours such as aggression, excitability, sleepiness, itchiness,
- pressing its head against a wall, walking around in circles, avoiding light,
- blindness,
- fits may occur.

Even for the same disease, the signs vary. Some animals get a severe form and die, but others get a mild form with fever and loss of appetite and recover. Around 50% of cases die. Surviving animals slowly recover over several weeks, but some have permanent brain damage or blindness.

How to prevent viral encephalomyelitis

Vaccines are available against EEE, WEE, VEE and are used in the USA. In Japan, horses (and people) are regularly vaccinated against JEE. There is no vaccine against WNE.

How to treat viral encephalomyelitis

As with any virus infection there is no specific treatment.

If the animal shows signs of changed behaviour:

- inject dexamethasone intramuscularly every six hours for two days, dose 0.05–0.1 mg per kg body weight, or
- inject flunixin meglumine intramuscularly every 12 hours, dose 0.5 mg per kg body weight.

If the animal has fits, keep it on soft ground to reduce injury. It can be treated initially with:

- diazepam (Vallium),
  - foal of 50 kg weight: 5–20 mg intravenously
  - adult horse 400 kg weight: 20–80 mg intravenously;
- or xylazine (Rompun),
  - foal of 50 kg weight: 25–50 mg intravenously
  - adult horse 400 kg weight: 250–400 mg intravenously.

11.8 Equine viral arteritis

The infection may occur worldwide, but many infections do not make the horse ill and are not noticed. Adult animals do not usually die from it, but young foals do.

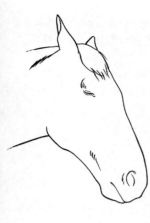

What EVA looks like

In some places the infection can cause the signs listed below and lead to death. In other places, infection may cause only mild illness that is hardly noticed.

- Fever up to 41°C (106°F),
- dull behaviour and stops eating,
- swelling (oedema) under the skin of the eyelids,
- blood-stained tears,
- swelling of the legs and belly,
- similar swellings may occur on the sides of the face and neck,
- discharge from the eyes and nose,
- pregnant mares may abort,
- sometimes a cough.

The disease can look similar to other conditions resulting in swellings on the body. Mild forms of EVA can look like infections that affect breathing, such as flu (see the section *Flu*), and so the signs do not easily identify it.

How to prevent EVA

In an outbreak, if possible avoid contact between sick and healthy horses.

Laboratory needed!

Confirmation of EVA is a job for specialized laboratories, which may find the virus in samples or may test blood samples for evidence of EVA. Where advanced laboratory facilities exist, infected animals are identified from samples taken and the positive animals are kept separate from others for at least one month.

A vaccine is available and is sometimes used in breeding animals in areas where EVA is a problem. Permission from the veterinary authorities may be required to use the vaccine.

How to treat EVA

There is no treatment effective against this disease, but inject antibiotics to protect against additional infections.

11.9 African horse sickness

Midge

This disease occurs in sub-Saharan Africa and has spread to Spain, Portugal, the Arab peninsular and the Indian subcontinent. Biting insects such as midges transmit it. It is believed that midges pick up the infection from zebras. The disease is seasonal. Big outbreaks can follow heavy rain, which favours the insects' reproduction.

What African horse sickness looks like

Different forms, which vary in severity, are seen. In Africa, local donkeys and horses can be affected so mildly that the infection is not noticed. However, mules and imported horses can get a severe infection and die. In all forms, there is a fever of 40°–41°C (105°–106°F).

The signs of the different forms of African horse sickness are as follows.

SEVEREST FORM

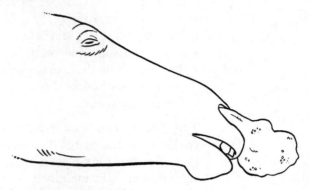

- Difficult breathing and coughing,
- the animal continues to eat,
- yellowish fluid and froth from the nose,
- sweating,
- the horse lies down,
- death four or five days after the first signs.

MILDER FORM

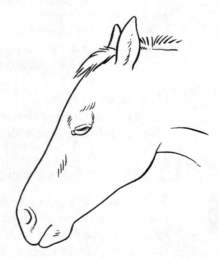

- Swelling (oedema) around the eyes and bulging of the inside of the eyelid,
- swollen lips,
- blood spots below the skin under the tongue,
- difficulty in swallowing,

- death does not always follow, but if the animal does die it happens up to two weeks after the first signs.

MIXED FORM
A mixture of the severest and milder forms can occur.

How to prevent African horse sickness
Vaccinate horses, donkeys or mules before they are transported to an affected area.

How to treat African horse sickness
- There is no treatment. Nursing care is all that can be provided in the hope that the horse will recover.
- Antibiotic injections, for example, penicillin with streptomycin, are given to protect against secondary infections.

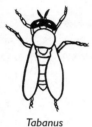

Tabanus

11.10 Equine infectious anaemia, swamp fever

This disease has been found in North and South America, Africa, Europe, Asia and Australia. Biting insects such as horse flies spread it.

What equine infectious anaemia looks like
- Temperature of 38.5°–40.5°C (101.3°–105°F).
- The animal goes off its food.
- Pregnant mares may abort.

Most animals recover after this stage. Often, owners do not notice that the horse has been ill. Some animals do not show any more signs, but others may show the following signs after two to three weeks:

- fever,
- weight loss,
- dull behaviour,
- small blood spots under the skin of mucous membranes,
- difficulty in walking,
- jaundice,
- swelling (oedema) of the lower belly,
- rapid pulse,
- weakness.

Most cases that show these signs die within one year. Up to that time:

- they become weaker,
- they periodically get a fever with blood spots again showing on the mucous membranes,
- towards the end the colour of the mucous membranes becomes pale.

How to prevent equine infectious anaemia

Biting insects, such as horse flies, spread it. Keep ill animals as far away as possible from others to reduce the chance of insects carrying the infection between them.

Vets may take a blood sample for a special test, called the Coggins test, to find out if an animal has had the illness.

Using the same surgical instruments or hypodermic needles without sterilizing them can spread the disease. Cases that have recovered from the disease look normal, but have the virus in their blood. Therefore, it is very important to sterilize instruments properly. See the section *How to sterilize equipment*.

Treatment

There is no effective treatment.

11.11   Nagana, African trypanosomiasis

Tsetse fly

This disease is caused by a microscopic *Trypanosoma* spp. parasite, which gets into the blood from an insect bite. In Africa, the tsetse fly is the insect that normally transmits it. Therefore, the disease is mainly found where tsetse flies live.

What African trypanosomiasis looks like

It is usually a slow disease with variable signs. The signs of trypanosomiasis may include:

- a fever that comes and goes,
- dull behaviour,
- the animal becomes tired easily and may stop eating,
- a discharge from the eye,
- swollen lymph nodes,
- pale mucous membranes (see the section *How to check mucous membranes*),
- becomes thinner and weaker over a period of weeks,
- swollen limbs and belly with oedema (see the chapter *Lumps under the skin* for how to recognize oedema),
- there may be signs that the brain is infected, for example, pressing the head against a wall, walking round in circles or paralysis.

The animal usually dies after two to four months.

Laboratory needed!

Usually the disease is identified when the small parasites are found in a blood sample, using a microscope. See the section *How to collect samples for laboratory tests* for how to make a sample of blood ready for microscopic examination. It is more likely that parasites will be found if the blood sample is taken when the animal has a fever. Later in the disease, fewer trypanosomes can be found in the blood.

How to prevent African trypanosomiasis

Control of the African tsetse fly is a major undertaking. It is normally carried out to make it possible to keep cattle on land that cannot otherwise be grazed by cattle because of this disease. There have been large-scale programmes, such as insecticidal sprays from aircraft, and local initiatives, such as insect traps.

The other approach to control is to inject the animals regularly with a drug that kills trypanosomes. This is usually done for cattle, not horses and donkeys. There is no vaccine.

How to treat African trypanosomiasis

Inject one of the following drugs according to the manufacturer's instructions:

- homidium bromide (Ethidium), dose 1 mg per kg body weight,
- quinapyramine sulphate (Antrycide), dose 5 mg per kg body weight.

Diminazene aceturate (Berenil) is not recommended for horses, so do not give it if alternative drugs are available. If there is no alternative, a suggested dose for Berenil is given for the disease dourine (see below).

11.12 Surra

Stomoxys

This is also a trypanosomiasis disease, but biting flies other than tsetse flies transmit the parasite that causes surra. It occurs in places where there are no tsetse flies, including North Africa, India, Southeast Asia, the Middle East and Latin America.

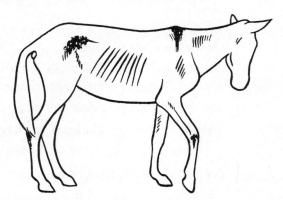

What surra looks like

- Wasting,
- fever that comes and goes,
- pale mucous membranes,
- oedema swellings of legs and belly,
- thinness,

- discharge from the eyes,
- there may be small blood spots on the pink skin (conjunctiva) inside the eyelids,
- in the later stages, the brain is affected. Then there may be fits or the animal may be weak on its hind legs and unable to walk properly.

Without treatment, surra always leads to death. This can happen after just a few days or after several months.

How to prevent surra

It is impossible to avoid bites from flies. There is no vaccine. Early identification and treatment is necessary. However, the risk of infection from the bite of a carrier fly can be reduced by using fly repellents (see the section *Flies*), and by treating wounds promptly.

How to treat surra

Some of the drugs that may be used to treat surra are given below.

QUINAPYRAMINE SULPHATE

Give a subcutaneous injection of quinapyramine sulphate (Antrycide), dose 3 mg per kg body weight. This can be toxic, so work out the total dose and give half in a first injection and the other half in a second injection six hours later.

ISOMETAMIDIUM CHLORIDE

Different manufacturers call this drug Trypamidium or Samorin. It is usually sold in a 1 g sachet.

To prepare a 2% solution, mix a 1 g sachet in 50 ml of boiled and cooled water.

Dose of isometamidium

A 2% solution is 2 g of medicine in 100 ml water,
which is 20 mg medicine in one ml of solution.

The dose is 0.5 mg of isometamidium per kg body weight.

Therefore, one ml of solution is for 40 kg body weight.

For a 100 kg animal, 2.5 ml of solution is needed.

For a 400 kg horse, 10 ml of solution is needed.

Give as an intramuscular injection. Split the dose and inject in several places and rub after injection.

DIMINAZENE ACETURATE

This drug is sold as Berenil. It is used, but it can be toxic to horses. Follow the manufacturer's instructions.

It is given by intramuscular injection. First give a dose of 7 mg per kg body weight, then give another injection of half this dose 24 hours later.

11.13 Dourine

The trypanosome that causes this disease is transmitted when horses or donkeys mate. The disease may occur in South America, Africa (particularly northern and southern Africa) and parts of Asia.

What dourine looks like
- Oedema (for how to identify oedema, see the chapter *Lumps under the skin*) of the skin around the penis or the lips of the vulva, which means the lips under the tail of the mare.
- Discharge from the penis or from the vagina of mares.
- The swelling spreads to the belly and enlarges.
- Oedema swellings appear on the sides of the body.
- Later on, thinness and weakness progress.
- Weakness on both hind legs.

About half of the animals with this disease die from it.

How to prevent dourine
Where the disease is established, mares may be treated with Berenil at the time of mating. A laboratory test on a serum sample can be used to identify infected animals.

How to treat dourine
This is never completely effective in all cases. Some animals recover, but remain as a source of infection to others. It is not recommended to treat dourine. Euthanasia is recommended.

Two drugs could be used to treat dourine, but both can be toxic:

- quinapyramine sulphate (Antrycide), which is used as for surra.
- diminazine (Berenil), see surra treatment for dose.

12 Colic, pain in the belly

Colic means pain in the digestive tract, that is, the stomach or intestines.

What colic looks like
- Restlessness,
- pawing the ground,
- kicking its belly,
- sweating.

Note that other events can cause these signs, for example, giving birth.

12.1 How to decide if the colic is likely to be serious

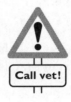

Call vet!

Diagnosis is complex and best left to a veterinarian if one is available.

Colic may be mild or serious. Without professional advice, it is sometimes possible to decide if the colic is likely to be serious by checking the pulse rate, the colour inside the eyelid and the breathing.

Pulse rate
The animal's pulse rate is a useful guide to how serious the colic is. See the chapter *How to check signs of a horse or donkey's health* for normal pulse rates and how to take the pulse. If the number of heart beats per minute is near normal, usually the colic is not serious.

Pulse rate and severity of colic

Pulse rate of the horse	Seriousness of colic
50 beats per minute or less	Not a serious colic
50–60	This is a sign of pain, but not too worrying
60–80	This is a worrying pulse rate, especially if it stays high after the horse is given a pain-killing drug
More than 80	Very serious; the horse may die or may need to be euthanased

Colour inside eyelid
The colour of the skin inside the eyelid is normally pink. It is a poor sign when the inside of the eyelid is a dull red colour ('brick red'),

or yellowish with little blood vessels clearly showing. If it looks purple, death is usually close.

Breathing

It is more likely to be serious colic if:
- the breathing is much faster than normal,
- the nostrils are wide open,
- the breathing sounds like sighing.

12.2   Causes, prevention and general care of colic

Some of the more common causes

FOOD
- Sudden change to what the horse eats,
- too much food, for example, if a horse eats too much grain from a sack,
- poor quality food, such as mouldy hay, or too much dry straw,
- long gaps between meals,
- fresh, highly fermentable green fodder that produces gas.

WATER
- Not enough clean drinking water,
- water not supplied regularly,
- rapid drinking of too much water.

INTERNAL PARASITES
- Red-worms have a developing stage that damages blood vessels to the gut.
- Bot larvae in excessive numbers may sometimes cause colic.

BAD TEETH
For example, if the back teeth have sharp edges the horse may not chew its food properly.

SAND
The animal may swallow sand if it is grazing on sandy ground where there is not much grass.

EATING STRANGE THINGS
For example, horses and donkeys sometimes eat plastic bags, or pieces of rope.

Prevention of colic
- Feed small quantities of good quality food at regular intervals.
- Do not prevent the horse from eating for a long period, and then let it eat a lot.

- Keep sacks of grain in a place where the horse cannot get to them.
- Make sure water is offered frequently during the day. Little and often is best, especially in hot climates.
- Remember that, if an animal does not have any food or water for a long time, it may over-eat or drink too much and then get a digestive problem.
- Advice on how to prevent internal parasites is given in the section on parasites.
- Make sure teeth are rasped regularly.

General care

- Try to get professional help from a vet if possible.
- Remove food until the colicky pain has stopped. Keep the animal somewhere without food and without bedding material it could eat. The first meal after recovery should be a small bran mash and a small amount of fresh green fodder.
- Give treatment for worms.
- Listen to the noises in the guts by pressing your ear against the horse's belly. Give appropriate treatment according to the signs of what kind of colic it is.

Signs of colic and appropriate treatment

Guts very noisy *and pulse rate* ➜ *Give treatment for spasmodic colic (colic with less than 60 beats per minute* | *gut muscle cramps)*

Very quiet guts or no sounds ➜ *Give treatment for colic because of blockage with impacted food*

Gassy 'ping' sounds ➜ *Give treatment for colic with a lot of gas*

12.3   Colic with gut muscle cramps, spasmodic colic

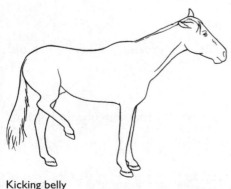
Kicking belly

What spasmodic colic looks like

The animal shows signs of pain that stop and start. These signs may be:

- rolling,
- sweating,
- kicking at the belly or stamping,

The pulse rate may go up to 50 beats per minute, but when the gut pain stops it goes back to normal after a few minutes.

How to treat spasmodic colic

Give an injection to relieve pain. For example, give hyoscine with dipyrone (Buscopan) by intravenous injection (if given by injection into the muscle, this drug may cause an abscess), or flunixin meglamine (Finadyne). See the *List of medicines* at the back of the book for doses.

These cases usually respond well to treatment for pain.

12.4   Colic with a lot of gas

This type of colic can follow eating a lot of fresh green food.

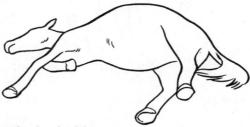

What gas colic looks like
- The belly is usually swollen with gas and there are sounds of gas gurgling and rumbling inside.
- The pain may stop and start.
- The pulse does not usually rise above about 50.

How to treat gas colic
- Give phenylbutazone by intravenous injection.
- Alternatively, give 1.1 mg per kg body weight flunixin meglamine (Finadyne) by intravenous or intramuscular injection.

These cases usually respond well to treatment for pain. These drugs reduce the pain, but do not stop the contractions of the gut muscles, which help the animal to get rid of the gas.

12.5   Colic because of blockage with impacted food

This kind of colic can occur after the animal has eaten a diet with a lot of dry straw. The food being digested can become stuck in a hard, dry mass in the latter parts of the guts, which are called the colon and caecum.

What impaction colic looks like
- The animal is not usually in as much pain as with colic with a lot of gas, but pain may become stronger over a few days.
- The horse may strain as though it wants to pass urine, holding its tail high.
- It may look round at its belly, scrape the ground with a front foot, or yawn.
- There are no loud noises of gas in the belly.

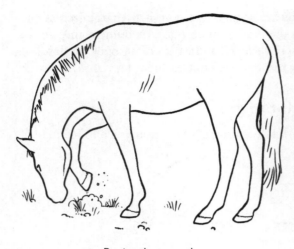

Pawing the ground

How to treat impaction colic

Give liquid paraffin by stomach tube. Liquid paraffin is a clear, oily fluid available from pharmacies and is *not* the same as paraffin for cooking stoves.

Give 2–4 litres of liquid paraffin (2 litres for a donkey or small pony, 4 litres for a large horse) twice a day for three days. Give the same amount of salt solution (7 g of salt per litre of water) at the same time.

It is best to give the fluid by stomach tube (see the section *How to use a stomach tube*). Alternatively, pour it into the corner of the animal's mouth using a funnel, but be sure to allow the animal plenty of time to swallow so that it does not choke.

12.6 Sand colic

This is a particular type of blockage of the intestines. It occurs in horses in desert environments where there is sandy ground and not much grass.

What sand colic looks like

Call vet!

- It is very painful. The horse may show signs of great pain, such as kicking its belly, rolling, sweating, and may have an anxious expression in its eye.
- Put a lump of the animal's dung in a jar of water, and mix it. In cases of sand colic, sand is likely to settle at the bottom of the jar.

Treatment is difficult. Surgery may be necessary, a job for an experienced veterinarian.

12.7 Colic with a twist in the gut

If the gut has twisted, pain is very strong. The horse will roll. Its pulse will be high and it will probably show other signs of serious colic.

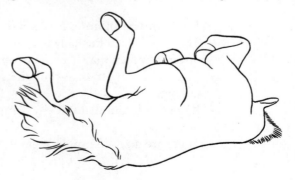

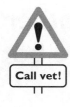

Call vet!

These cases can usually only be cured by surgery carried out by an experienced vet. Even with an operation, not all survive.

If a horse had great pain but continues to have a very high pulse after giving injections to relieve pain, its chances of surviving are poor. Following a twist in the gut, the blood supply to part of the gut is stopped, and that part of the gut dies. Then gut contents leak out inside the horse. After the strong pain stops, the horse may start sweating, or just stand and shiver. This is a poor sign.

Other poor signs are:

- The pulse rate is above 80 beats per minute.
- There are more than 40 breaths per minute.
- The skin under the eyelids looks purple or black.
- Foul-smelling fluid may come down the nose.
- The body temperature is low (for example, 36°C).

When you see these poor signs, the kindest action may be euthanasia. See the chapter *How to shoot a horse*.

12.8   Food stuck in the neck, choke

Sometimes dry food, for example, some pelleted food, swells with the animal's saliva and gets stuck after being swallowed.

What choke looks like
- Drooling saliva.
- If the animal tries to swallow, chewed food or water may come down the nose.
- The animal is distressed.
- It may be possible to feel the blockage in the neck.

How to prevent choke
Soak dried food in water before feeding it.

How to treat choke
- Do not give food or water.
- Most cases do not need any treatment, but it may take several hours for the blockage to pass.
- Very carefully pass a stomach tube (see the section *How to use a stomach tube*).
- Drugs to stop muscle spasm may be useful, for example, hyoscine with dipyrone (Buscopan).

13 Diarrhoea, worms and other parasites living inside the body

13.1 Diarrhoea of adults

What causes diarrhoea of adults

In many cases the reason for diarrhoea is not found out. Some of the causes are:

1 stress,
2 food, for example:
   - a sudden change of diet (such as, a lot of fresh grass, or too much grain),
   - mouldy food,
3 parasitic worms,
4 infections, which may cause blood-stained diarrhoea,
5 eating sand,
6 tumour (cancer) affecting the gut,
7 allergy.

Diarrhoea can be caused by *Salmonella*, which can make people very sick. After handling or treating any animal with diarrhoea, always wash your hands carefully with soap.

How to treat diarrhoea of adult animals

- Fluids. All cases with diarrhoea should be encouraged to drink as much as possible. Offer the animal a mixture of:

  4 litres of clean water
  8 heaped tablespoons of sugar
  1 heaped teaspoon of salt

  Mix fresh each day, and throw away what has not been drunk after 24 hours. If the animal is too weak to drink, liquid can be given by stomach tube. See the section *How to use a stomach tube*.

- Wash the diarrhoea off the skin and hair around the tail. Bandage the tail to help keep it clean.
- Keep the sick animal away from others.
- Give natural yoghurt. This can be given by stomach tube.
- Targetted treatment. If you are able to, decide the possible cause and give a treatment appropriate for it.

Treatment of diarrhoea in adult animals

Cause	How to treat or prevent
Stress	Remove stress
Change of diet	Make changes slowly over a period of several days
Mouldy food	Replace with fresh food
Worms	Treat with anthelminthic (see sections about worms)
Infections	If there is fever, antibiotic injections may be useful
Sand	Graze animals away from sandy places; provide alternative food
Tumour	No effective treatment exists, so euthanasia may be appropriate
Allergy	Avoid access to the allergen, for example, mouldy food

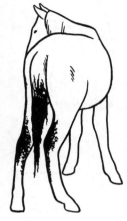

ANTIBIOTIC INJECTIONS

Antibiotics do not help cure most types of diarrhoea, even those caused by infection. In fact, it is believed that sometimes antibiotics cause colitis, which results in diarrhoea.

Antibiotics suitable for injection when an animal has diarrhoea caused by an infection are sulphonamides or penicillin-streptomycin or ampicillin.

13.2   Diarrhoea of foals

Causes of diarrhoea of foals

1 Mother in heat (about ten days after birth and again three weeks later).
2 Parasitic worms.
3 Infections.

How to treat and prevent diarrhoea of foals

- Mix the same solution as described for adults and encourage the foal to drink as much as possible,
- keep the foal warm,
- decide the likely cause and give a treatment appropriate for it.

Treatment of diarrhoea in foals

Cause	Treatment
Mare in heat	No treatment necessary because the diarrhoea will pass when the mare is no longer in heat
Worms	Treat with medicine to kill worms (see later in this chapter)
Infections	If the foal has a fever, give antibiotic injections (see note above on antibiotic use for diarrhoea of adults)

13.3 The life stories of worms

There are variations with different kinds of worms, but the basic life stories of roundworms and tapeworms are given below.

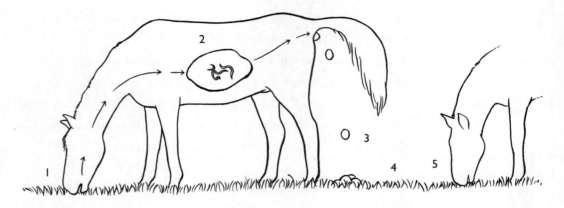

Life cycles of roundworms and tapeworms

Roundworm life story	Stage	Tapeworm life story
Tiny roundworm larvae are accidentally eaten with grass	1	Tapeworm larvae inside forage mites are accidentally eaten
The young worms move around in the animal's body The worms feed in the guts and they lay eggs Lung worms feed in the lungs, but their eggs are swallowed and go through the guts	2	The tapeworms grow in the guts and they produce eggs
Roundworm eggs come out in the dung	3	The end of the tapeworm containing eggs drops off and comes out in the dung
Eggs hatch and develop into tiny larvae and most die in the grass	4	Mites in the grass eat some eggs and they develop into tapeworm larvae inside the mites
Some new roundworm larvae are accidentally eaten	5	Some new tapeworm larvae are accidentally eaten with a mouthful of grass

13.4 Red-worm disease (strongylosis)

Red-worms are found worldwide. The larvae cause colic and death. The different species vary in length from about 20 to 50 mm.

What red-worm disease looks like

Red-worms cause two kinds of disease. The young worms moving around the animal's body cause one type. This can result in:

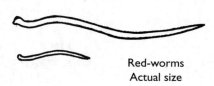

Red-worms
Actual size

- pain and colic,
- fever,
- loss of appetite,
- sudden death from internal bleeding (due to damage to an artery to the intestine).

Adult worms attach to the inside of the guts and feed on the animal's blood. This results in:

- weakness and poor body condition,
- pale mucous membranes.

How to prevent red-worm disease

- Dose with deworming medicine two to four times per year. Ready-filled syringes to squirt into the mouth are popular in rich countries. Suitable drugs are listed at the back of the book.
- If the animals live in a fenced place, pick up the dung and remove it. It is best to do this daily, but removing it twice weekly can be effective. Worm eggs are removed with the dung, so there will be fewer larvae on the land to infect the horses.
- Deworming does not have to be done so often if dung is removed. For example, in places with a cold winter deworm at the beginning of summer and again after two months. In places with a hot climate and a rainy season, deworm at the end of the dry season and again after two months.

How to treat red-worm disease

There is no effective treatment for serious damage by larvae to the arteries that take blood to the intestines. At an earlier stage, treat with a worm medicine effective against larvae, for example, iver-mectin or fenbendazole (Panacur).

13.5 Large roundworms (ascarid worms)

This worm is a problem for young foals, but does not normally cause disease in adults, which acquire immunity. The worms live in the intestine.

What ascarid worm disease looks like

Heavy infections with these worm cause:

- coughing,
- weakness and thinness,

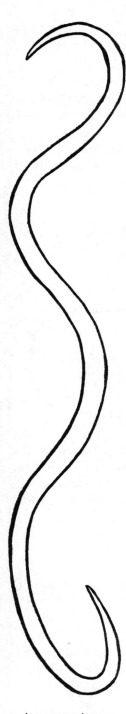

Large roundworm
(ascarid worm)
Actual size

- the foal eats, but does not grow well
- large, white worms are sometimes seen in the foal's dung.

If a dung sample is taken to a laboratory, worm eggs should be seen with a microscope.

How to prevent ascarid worm disease
- Eggs produced by worms in the foals can remain on the ground and be infective the following year, so, if possible, keep mares and foals on different ground the next year.
- Treat all foals when eight weeks old. This is sufficient time for the foal's immunity to develop, but is not enough time for generations of the worm to mature, produce eggs and re-infest the foal.

How to treat ascarid worm disease
Use any of the medicines for roundworms listed in the back of the book. Piperazine or ivermectin are very effective.

13.6 Tapeworms

Tapeworm
Actual size
Some species are bigger and others are much smaller

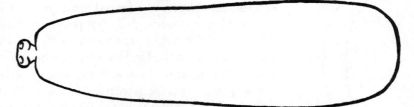

These worms are not as harmful to horses as roundworms. The ones found in horses may look different from those found in other animals, or in humans. They live in the large intestine and may be up to 80 cm long, depending on the species of tapeworm. More often they are less than 20 cm long.

What tapeworm disease looks like
- There are usually no signs of infection.
- Large numbers of tapeworms may help cause blockage in the gut and colic.

How to treat tapeworm disease
Drugs for roundworms are not effective. It is possible to use pyrantel (Strongid P). See the list of medicines at the back of the book.

13.7 Bots, Gasterophilus larvae

These are the maggots of flies, which lay eggs on the hairs of horses and donkeys, often on the front legs, neck or face. The horse or

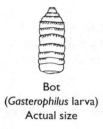

Bot
(*Gasterophilus* larva)
Actual size

donkey swallows the eggs when it licks its coat. The bots live inside the stomach.

Sometimes bots can be seen attached just inside the back passage when the horse passes its dung. One type of bot reattaches here for a few days just before leaving the horse's body to develop into the adult fly. Bots are sometimes seen in the dung. At post-mortem examination it is common to see groups of them attached inside the stomach.

Bots are not thought to cause serious disease. Where the eggs first hatch tiny maggots may irritate the skin, especially around the lips. Older bots can damage the lining of the stomach, leading to ulcers.

Bots can be treated with ivermectin or organophosphorus drugs. See the list at the back of the book.

13.8 Pinworm (*Oxyuris*)

Causes itchiness under the tail. See the chapter *Diseases and parasites of the skin*.

13.9 Lung worms

See the chapter *Diseases affecting breathing*.

13.10 Liver fluke disease

Liver fluke
Actual size

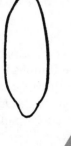

The fluke is a leaf-shaped parasite that lives in the tubes (bile ducts) of the liver. It causes disease more severely and more frequently in cattle, sheep and goats than horses.

What liver fluke disease looks like
Flukes are believed to sometimes cause tiredness, loss of appetite and swellings (oedema) on the skin. There are no signs unique to the disease.

Experienced laboratory workers may find fluke eggs in a dung sample looked at with a microscope. See the section *How to collect samples for laboratory tests*.

Laboratory
needed!

How to prevent liver fluke disease
Animals become infected when eating leaves in swampy areas, so avoid grazing these places if flukes are a problem.

How to treat liver fluke disease
Oxyclozanide (Zanil) or triclabendazole (Fasinex) are used to treat fluke in cattle and can be used for horses.

13.11 Leech

When a horse or donkey drinks, a leech living in the water will sometimes attach to the inside of the mouth. Leeches may stay attached for several hours as they engorge on the animal's blood.

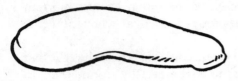

Leech
Actual size
Size varies with different species, and before and after feeding on blood.

What leeches look like
- The first sign that a leech has attached may be blood in the animal's mouth.
- Hold the tongue and look inside the mouth, including under the tongue. A dark red leech may be seen.

How to treat leeches
Carefully pull the leech off. The wound may bleed for some time after removing the leech, because leeches produce chemicals that slow down blood clotting. However, the wounds rarely become infected and no other treatment is necessary.

13.12 Hydatid disease

The hydatid is the larva of a small dog or fox tapeworm called *Echinococcus granulosus*. The dog gets the worm when it eats meat containing the tapeworm larvae. This may be sheep, cattle or pig meat or horse or donkey meat, especially offal such as the liver and lungs. In horses, the liver is where the larvae, called 'hydatids', are most commonly found.

Hydatid disease is serious for people, so if you suspect it in animals, try to get advice from a medical worker about how to protect people from it.

What hydatid disease looks like
It is usually only seen after a horse has died: the liver and lungs in particular may have bubble-like growths with a whitish capsule. These cysts may be the size of tennis balls, or as large as 20 cm across. They have clear liquid inside. This liquid contains small, white specks.

Treatment
There is no treatment for hydatid disease in horses and donkeys.

Dogs should be treated with a medicine effective against the tapeworm, for example, praziquantel. People should always wash their hands very carefully with soap immediately after touching dogs that may carry this tapeworm.

14 Thin animals, liver disease and diseases causing urine problems

14.1 Thin animals

Horses and donkeys become weak and thin when they use more energy than they get in their diet. This can have many causes. Some of the important ones are shown in the table.

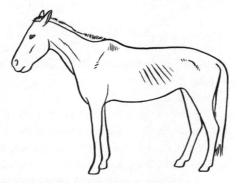

Thin animals: causes and treatment

What makes horses and donkeys thin	How to treat the problem
Not enough food	➜ Give more food
Not enough energy in the food, for example, too much straw and not enough grain	➜ Add some high quality food to the diet ➜ Carbohydrates are a good source of energy; for example, starch in grains (such as oats, sorghum, or barley) or raw cane sugar (called *jaggery* in India) ➜ Fats, such as vegetable cooking oil, are a very good source of energy; a cup of cooking oil can be added to each feed; linseed or rapeseed oil can be given
Not a mixed, balanced diet, for example, only chopped dry straw or chaff (*boussa*)	➜ Give some fresh green food as well ➜ Make sure there is also enough energy in the food ➜ Young horses fed only bran may get problems with bone growth causing a swollen head; this is caused by the wrong balance of calcium in this food

Bad teeth	→ Check teeth; rasp if necessary (see section *Tooth rasping*)
Worms	→ Treat (see chapter about worms and the list of drugs at the back of the book)
Too much work	→ Reduce the work, give more time to rest, lighten the load → Allow more time to graze
Slowly developing liver disease	→ See next section
Other disease, such as chronic infection or cancerous growths	→ Try to work out what kind of disease it is → Refer to appropriate section of the book for suggested treatment or ask for help from a veterinarian

Advice for feeding a thin, sick horse

- If a starved horse is fed too much too quickly, it may get diarrhoea and colic.
- Therefore, feed small amounts often.
- Gradually increase the amount of food each day.
- Give 0.75–1 kg of grain five or six times per day.
- Take away food that has not been eaten after two hours.
- For animals with a poor appetite, encourage feeding by offering fresh, green leaves, such as alfalfa, or molasses. Hay should be fresh, not old, dusty or mouldy.
- Thin horses will benefit from the energy in vegetable cooking oil. Add it to the feed, making a total of up to 0.5 litre per day.

14.2 Liver disease

Liver disease may happen suddenly or develop slowly. Liver disease is quite common in horses and often causes death.

Poisonous plants, chemicals eaten by the horse or infections can all cause sudden liver disease. Arsenic and lead are examples of chemicals that damage the liver.

What sudden liver disease looks like

- Animal stops eating,
- constipation usually,
- dark-coloured urine,
- behaves in a dull manner,
- may stand with half-eaten hay hanging from its mouth,
- in most cases the mucous membranes have a yellowish colour (jaundice), but jaundice does not always mean liver disease,

- photosensitization (see the section *Sunburn, photosensitization*) sometimes causing oozing cracks on the lips and muzzle and a blue-grey colour to affected skin,

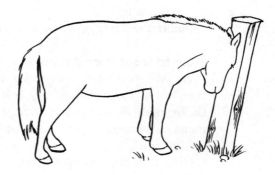

- sometimes, in the most severe cases, strange behaviour such as:
  - walking round in circles or wandering aimlessly,
  - pressing head against a wall,
  - mad excitement,
  - fits.

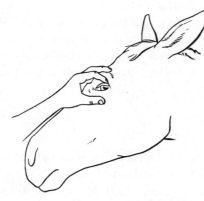

A NOTE ABOUT JAUNDICE

Yellowish mucous membranes (see the section *How to check the mucous membranes*) are a common sign in liver disease.

However, some animals have mucous membranes that always look a bit jaundiced, especially Arab horses, grey horses and donkeys. Any horse that has not eaten for a few days can look mildly jaundiced. Do not assume that yellow colour of the mucous membranes always means liver disease.

How to prevent sudden liver disease

Avoid access to known poisonous plants or to poisonous chemicals, such as old car batteries containing lead.

The cause of slowly developing (chronic) liver disease may be poisoning by plants in the *Senecio* family, such as ragwort.

What slowly developing liver disease looks like

- Slow loss of weight,
- pale mucous membranes,
- loss of appetite,
- weakness and unsteady walk,
- swelling (oedema) under the belly,
- photosensitization,

- eventually, in the most serious cases,
  - yawning,
  - pressing head against a wall or tree,
  - standing with food in mouth,
  - staggering,
- finally, the horse goes down to the ground and dies.

How to treat liver disease

Even with treatment, many cases of severe liver disease do not survive. Milder cases of sudden liver disease can be treated. However, if the animal shows signs of strange behaviour, such as mad excitement, euthanasia is recommended.

- Give the animal complete rest.
- Keep it out of sunlight.
- Feed hay and avoid foods with more protein, such as alfalfa or manufactured pellets. Add glucose to the diet.
- Encourage the animal to drink well.
- If it does not drink, give liquid by stomach tube (see the section *How to use a stomach tube*). It is best to give a salt solution. A recipe is given in the section *Diarrhoea of adults*.
- Give multivitamin injections containing B vitamins and vitamin K.
- If constipated, give 500 ml liquid paraffin (*not* kerosene or paraffin fuel) by stomach tube. Repeat once daily as necessary.
- Antibiotic injections, such as trimethoprim-sulphadiazine, dose 15–30 mg per kg body weight.

14.3 Red urine

Urine problems are rare with horses. Horse urine is usually cloudy and rarely clear. Cloudy urine does not indicate disease.

Urine may be red because it has blood in it. It may also be red because a disease has damaged the red blood cells, and the red pigment from blood has dissolved in the urine. To tell the difference, collect some red urine in a small bottle. Put the bottle where it will not be moved and leave it for 30 minutes. If it contains red blood cells, the red colour is stronger at the bottom of the bottle. If the urine has red pigment in it, the red colour stays evenly in the whole sample.

Diseases which can cause blood in urine

- Kidney infection,
- heavy infestation with red-worms (the larvae occasionally get into the kidneys),
- bladder infection,
- stones in the bladder,

- stones in the tube leading from the bladder to the outside (not usually a problem of females).

Diseases which can cause red pigment in the urine
- Equine infectious anaemia.
- Babesiosis.

14.4 Kidney and bladder infections

What kidney infection looks like
- Blood and pus in the urine,
- fever,
- loss of appetite,
- pain in the belly,
- weight loss.

What bladder infection looks like
- Blood and pus in the urine,
- often passes small amounts of urine,
- pain when passing urine,
- stands stretched out.

How to treat kidney or bladder infection
- Antibiotic injections. Use penicillin or sulphonamides. Treat for two weeks.
- Encourage the animal to drink water.

14.5 Stones in the urine

What the disease looks like
- Usually occurs in a male animal,
- often tries to pass urine, but the tube may be blocked,
- blood in urine,
- straining to pass urine,
- sometimes stones may be felt under the skin, beneath the tail, below the anus.

How to prevent stones in urine
Always give working animals enough clean water to drink. Offer water to them every few hours.

How to treat stones in urine
If an animal has this problem, treatment by a trained vet is needed.

A veterinarian may squirt saline in through a catheter to flush the penis and give an injection of a smooth muscle relaxant, which may help the animal to pass the stones.

Call vet!

15 Birth and care of foals

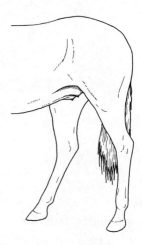

15.1 Normal birth

Most births occur at night and when the mare thinks she is not being watched.

One month before
- Swelling of the udder occurs from three to six weeks before foaling.

One day before
- Droplets of colostrum (first milk) usually appear on the nipples 6–48 hours before birth.

Four hours before
- The mare becomes restless and appears to have colic (kicks belly, swishes her tail, is unrelaxed).
- She wants to find a place on her own.
- She sweats at the shoulders and sides.

Birth (usually takes 10–30 minutes)
- Watery fluid pours out of the birth canal.
- The mare strains powerfully and usually lies down.
- A bag of fluid appears under the mare's tail with the foal's front feet inside it.

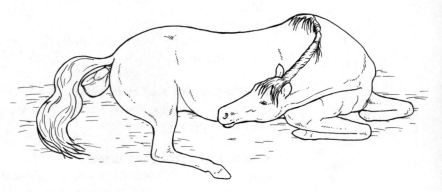

- The bag breaks, the head and body of the foal are pushed out and the foal takes its first breaths.

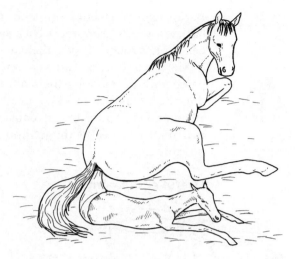

Note: Do not tie or break the umbilical cord because blood flows along it into the foal's body – wait for it to break naturally. The foal will be stronger if you do not break or cut the cord.

The 'afterbirth' (usually takes 30 minutes to 3 hours)

The mare continues to strain until the afterbirth (placenta) comes out. She does not normally eat it.

15.2   Helping with difficult births

If forceful straining by the mare has continued for several hours, there is probably a problem. The foetus may not be coming normally. It is normal for a foal to be born with its two front feet first followed by its head and shoulders. If any other parts of the body come first, birth is difficult.

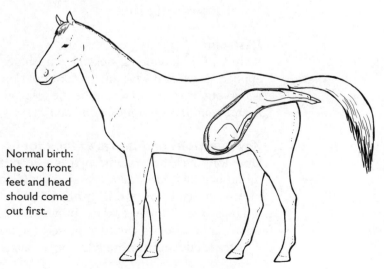

Normal birth: the two front feet and head should come out first.

Normally the foetus comes out in an upright position, that is, its back is towards its mother's back and its belly is towards its mother's belly. If it is rotated inside, there may not be a normal birth.

Mares' contractions are very strong and there is little time (compared with calves) after the main contractions start before the foal must be out and take its first breath. In problem births, the foal usually dies. Difficult births are dangerous for the mare. This is not an easy matter to deal with: get immediate professional advice if you possibly can.

Call vet!

Useful equipment

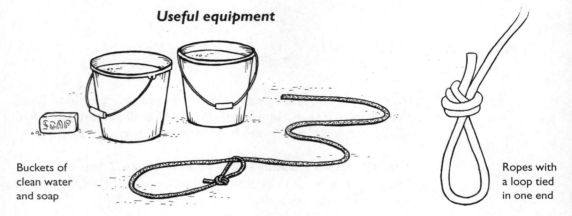

Buckets of
clean water
and soap

Ropes with
a loop tied
in one end

Getting ready to help with a difficult birth
1 Make sure you do not have long fingernails.
2 Take off any watch or jewellery on your hands or wrists.
3 Bandage the tail so that hairs do not get in the way.
4 Ask an assistant to hold the tail aside.
5 Wash around the lips of the birth canal with soap and water.
6 With clean water, wash hands and arms. Make your arms slippery with lots of soapy lather.

Restraint
Reduce the risk of being kicked by the mare. If she is a quiet animal, apply a twitch and have an assistant hold up a front leg. If the mare is nervous, cast the mare and tie the feet. See the chapter *How to tie, restrain and transport horses and donkeys.*

Key questions and things to look for
How long has the mare been trying to push out the foal? If it is more than 24 hours and the straining has stopped, most of the slippery fluid that helps normal birth will be lost.

Look to see if there is a dark, brown discharge. This is a sign that a very delayed case has started to putrefy (go rotten) inside the mother.

Is there any injury around the birth canal? Look for tearing.

Putting your hand inside

Put an arm inside. What can you feel? For example, are there:

- one or two feet?
- neck with mane, or ears, or mouth?
- no legs or head?
- twisted folds in the birth canal?

How to decide by feel if feet are front ones or back ones

The front leg has the knee above the fetlock joint, but the back leg has the angled hock joint above it. The fetlock joint and the joint above it bend the same way on a front leg, but on the hind leg, the hock joint above the fetlock bends the other way.

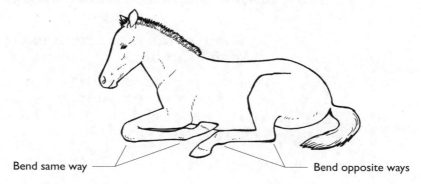

Bend same way ———— ———— Bend opposite ways

Try to work out which parts of the foal's body are coming first

Decide if it is coming normally, or not. If not, the aim is to try to move the head and two front feet to the normal position and then pull out the foal.

How to put ropes on the foetus

The loop at the end of the rope can be attached like this:

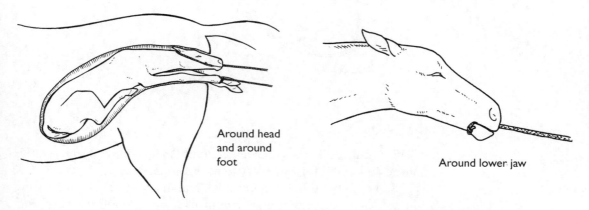

Around head
and around
foot

Around lower jaw

After using, ropes should be washed well and boiled or soaked in antiseptic, such as Savlon solution.

Lubrication

It is very much harder to pull out a dry foal than one which is still wet from the liquid which surrounds the foetus before birth. It helps a lot to introduce warm, clean, soapy water with a funnel and tube. Also, be sure your hands and arms are wet and slippery (with soap) before putting them inside the mare.

Oxytocin

Get trained helper!

Once you are sure that a foal is coming the right way, the mare may push it out with contractions of the uterus muscle without needing much pulling on the ropes.

If the contractions stop, experienced operators may give oxytocin slowly, by injection, to induce these contractions.

15.3 Some of the more common types of difficult birth

Call vet!

DIFFICULT BIRTHS ARE NORMALLY A JOB FOR A QUALIFIED VETERINAR-IAN. IF THERE IS NO ALTERNATIVE BUT FOR YOU TO HELP, TAKE GREAT CARE (1) NOT TO BE KICKED BY THE MARE, AND (2) NOT TO CAUSE UNNECESSARY SUFFERING TO THE MARE.

Head back

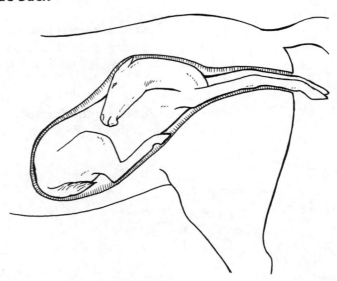

This is difficult because the neck is long, so it is difficult to reach the head and pull it forwards. Try to get veterinary help.

Sometimes, in the case of a small foal in a small horse or donkey, it may be possible to put an arm inside, cup it round the nose, and pull the head forward. At the same time, push the foal's shoulder back with your other hand.

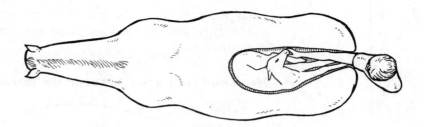

The foal lies across the birth canal (ventro-transverse presentation)

This is also very difficult to sort out. Feel up the feet to make sure it is not a case of twins. It is important to get veterinary help if you can. The vet will use anaesthetics to stop the mare from straining to push out the foetus while the operator is pushing legs back in.

If the mare is exhausted, and not straining, there is a chance of helping to deliver the foal. Cast the mare, tie her feet together (see the section *How to restrain horses and donkeys*), and turn her onto her back. To help to turn the foetus it is necessary to replace the lost foetal fluids in the mare with warm, clean soapy water.

Attach ropes to the two back feet of the foetus. Get an assistant to gently pull these while you push the head and front feet back inside the mare. Now pull the foal out back legs first.

Dog-sitting position

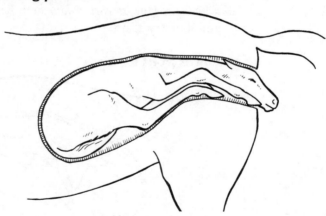

At first this case looks normal: the head and two front feet are coming. When you put your arm in the birth canal, you will feel the hind feet on the floor of it. If the owner of the horse has been pulling the head and two legs, and the mare has been straining, the foetus may be firmly stuck.

If the head and front feet are already out of the mare, the only way to get the foetus out is to cut it into pieces. This is a job for a veterinary surgeon, who will anaesthetize the mare.

If the case is not so advanced, use lots of soapy water in the birth

!
Call vet!

canal. Push the foetus back so the hind feet can be pushed back inside. Then pull the head and front feet out to deliver the foal in the normal position.

Head and neck down between the forelegs

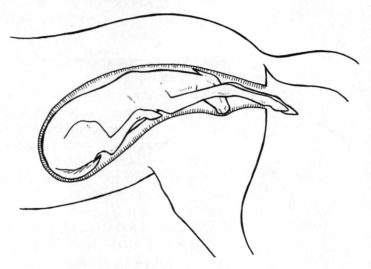

Put a rope loop around the lower jaw. Get an assistant to pull this while you push back on the forehead of the foetus.

If this does not work, tie the mare's feet together (see *How to cast a horse* or *How to cast a donkey* in Chapter 1), roll her on her back and then try again.

Lower front leg back

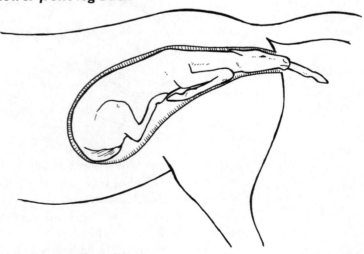

Push back the foetus' shoulder at the same time as bringing its foot forward. Cup the foot in your hand while you pull it, to protect the womb from injury.

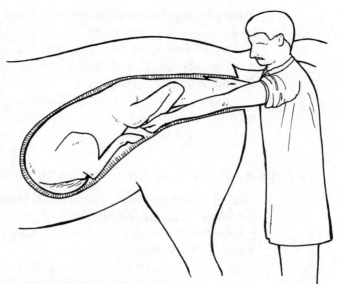

Whole front leg back

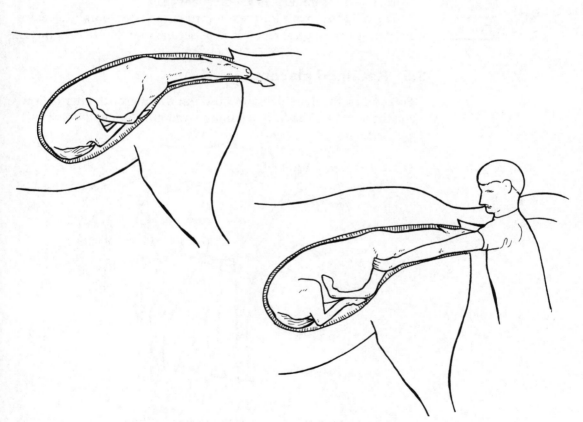

When the foetus is already dead, it may be necessary to cut off its head before bringing the rest of it out. Then, push it backwards, reach inside and pull the leg forwards.

Twisted pregnant womb (uterine torsion)

If, when you reached inside the birth canal when examining the case, spiral folds were felt in the wall, it suggests that the foal inside the womb has revolved inside the mare. These spirals show which way the womb has twisted.

Try to get your hand through the twisted folds to the foetus, hold on to a leg, and twist it in the opposite direction to the folds. The foal cannot be born while the womb is twisted.

15.4 Tearing around the birth canal

During a birth, the powerful contractions can lead to injury around the birth canal. Sometimes the foot of a foetus is pushed through the roof of the birth canal into the back passage down which the mare passes its dung.

Call vet!

Later there can be problems with dirty material causing infection of the vagina and womb. In most cases the animal can continue to work, but she is unlikely to get pregnant again.

The only treatment for these injuries is an operation by a veterinary surgeon. Surgical repair is done several months after the birth.

15.5 Retained placenta

Sometimes, the mare does not push out the afterbirth after delivering the foal. This can lead to laminitis and infection in the womb.

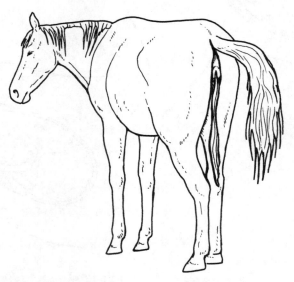

Leave alone for 24 hours. If the mare continues to be well in herself (eating, normal temperature and pulse rate), do nothing. Usually, it will come out in the next 24 hours with some foul-smelling, bloody fluid.

If the mare is not well, the placenta should be removed by hand. Wash your hands and arms very well. Have an assistant hold the tail to one side. Make sure the mare is restrained so that you cannot be kicked: get someone to hold a front leg up and have someone else apply a twitch if necessary.

With one hand, twist what hangs out of the back of the mare into a kind of rope. Put the other hand inside the mare and carefully move your fingers between the placenta and the wall of the womb to separate the two. Do not pull hard (or the womb may be pulled out – see the section *Prolapse of the uterus* below). When it is all separated, it should all come out.

If the mare has a raised temperature, and is not well, give antibiotic injections for three days.

15.6 Mastitis

Mastitis is caused by infection in the mammary gland or breast tissue of the mare. It is not common in horses and donkeys.

What mastitis looks like
- The mammary gland is hot and tender.
- Swelling (oedema) often develops in front of the gland.
- The mare may be ill, off her food and have a fever.

How to treat mastitis
Gently milk out the teats. Remove as much as possible (it may not look like normal milk) and repeat once an hour if possible.

Give antibiotic injections, for example, streptomycin with penicillin or trimethoprim with sulphonamides.

Tubes of antibiotic are used for cows with mastitis: the contents are squirted into the mammary gland. These tubes can be used in mares. Follow the instructions on the tube. However, the mare has several openings in the teat, unlike the cow, and the openings are smaller than a cow's. Only use tubes with a thin nozzle.

15.7 Hypocalcaemia, eclampsia, transit tetany

Hypocalcaemia means low calcium in the blood. Calcium is needed for normal muscle action. The condition can occur in mares producing milk or in any horses after transporting.

What hypocalcaemia looks like
- Sweating,
- stiff legs,
- twitching of muscles,
- the animal does not pass dung or urine.

The third eyelid is not across the eye, as in tetanus, which also causes stiff legs and muscle tremors.

Animals mildly affected after transport often recover without treatment. However, more seriously affected cases and mares producing milk go down after about 24 hours. Without treatment these cases may die two days after the illness started.

How to treat hypocalcaemia

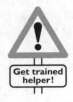

Give calcium borogluconate solution by slow injection into the jugular vein. The solution is usually used at 20% and the quantity needed is around 500 ml. It is given to effect: this means, give it slowly until the signs of hypocalcaemia start to disappear. This treatment usually results in complete recovery within about an hour.

15.8 Prolapse of back passage (rectum)

Part of the end of the tube which dung passes through may turn out of the body during birth. It normally goes back inside when the birth has completed.

If it does not go back, starve the mare for one to two days. Lubricate the rectum using water-soluble gel (KY Jelly) or very soapy water. Carefully push it back inside.

A serious case can develop if it has stayed outside for a long time and/or the attachments holding it inside were damaged during birth. If the part of the back passage tube that sticks out becomes a dark, purplish colour, there will be little chance of saving the life of the mare.

15.9 Prolapse of the uterus

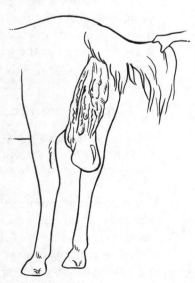

This condition, when the womb turns inside out after a birth and hangs down below the tail, is rare in horses and donkeys. When it occurs, there is usually tearing of internal blood vessels and internal bleeding. Mares often die if the uterus prolapses.

If it occurs, stand the mare facing down a slope, and wash any dirt off the womb. Then, push the womb back inside her.

If she struggles, for safety, tie her feet together, and roll her on her back to replace the organ (see the section *How to restrain horses and donkeys*). Again, try to find a place so her head is downhill from her tail.

15.10 Care of newborn foals

How to prevent foal diseases

THE FIRST MILK, COLOSTRUM

It is very important to make sure that, before it is 8–12 hours old, the foal drinks its mother's milk. This milk, called colostrum, contains antibodies that pass from the foal's stomach to its blood. Like temporary vaccination, the antibodies protect the foal from diseases.

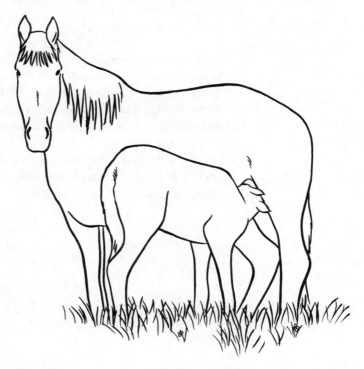

If the foal is unable to suck, gently milk the mare into a bucket. Pour this into a bottle and feed the foal from the bottle. To make a teat, put a condom with a hole in it on the end of the bottle. Give 500 ml at a time. Feed once per hour until the foal has had a total of 1–2 litres of colostrum.

Make sure that the floor where the newborn foal is kept is clean. There should be clean bedding, such as straw, from when it is first born. If the floor is dirty, it is more likely that the foal will get infection in its umbilical cord. This infection can enter the blood and cause joint-ill.

Diarrhoea
See the section *Diarrhoea of foals* in the chapter *Diarrhoea, worms and other parasites living inside the body*.

Failure to produce dung, retained meconium
Meconium is a substance that forms in the intestine during the foal's life in the womb. It is normally passed in the womb or as the first, hard dung after the foal is born. However, the meconium can be very hard and can cause a blockage.

WHAT RETAINED MECONIUM LOOKS LIKE
The foal may crouch and keep straining with its tail up as it tries to pass dung. It may be possible to feel hard material with a finger in the back passage of the foal.

HOW TO TREAT RETAINED MECONIUM
- Put a 10 cm piece of plastic tube from an old intravenous drip on the end of a 20 ml syringe, where the needle would go.
- Fill the syringe with liquid paraffin (this is not kerosene, but is a clear, oily liquid) or castor oil. If neither of these are available, use warm, soapy water.
- *Very* carefully, insert the tube into the rectum of the foal and slowly inject the oily liquid. The wall of the rectum of foals is not tough. Be careful not to damage it.

16 Eye problems

16.1 The healthy eye

How to prevent eye problems

- Every day wash around the eyes with a clean, wet cloth. This helps to get dust and dirt out of the eyes.
- Control flies and/or use fly repellent (see the chapter *Diseases and parasites of the skin* for advice on controlling flies).
- Use a fly fringe.

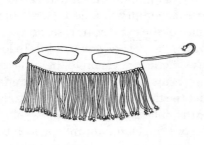
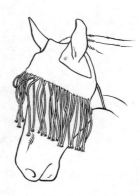

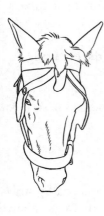

- If blinkers (blinders) are used on nervous, working horses in towns make sure that they are fitted properly and do not bang against the eye when the horse is trotting.

16.2 Injuries of eyelids

The eyelids are commonly injured. Sometimes they become bruised and swollen. More serious injuries also happen, in which the eyelids are torn.

How to treat eyelid injuries

BRUISING

- Bathe the area around the eyes with cotton wool soaked in cold, clean water.

CUTS

- If the eyelid is torn, when it heals the wound may contract. Therefore, it is better that these wounds are stitched when the wound is less than six hours old. Get help from a veterinarian if possible.

- Put antibiotic eye ointment into the eye.
- Make a fly fringe for the horse to keep insects from landing on the wound.

16.3 Things in the eye

Horses and donkeys may get pieces of hay or straw, insects or other things in their eyes. The object may get stuck under the third eyelid.

What the affected side looks like
- Eyelids closed,
- swollen eyelids,
- more tears.

How to treat it
1 Examine the eye.

Get a helper to hold the animal's head firmly. Look carefully in the eye for any injury or object. Hard objects like grit can scratch the surface of the eye (see next section).

Things in the eye are very painful. To look properly, drip special local anaesthetic for eyes on to the surface of the eye. Wait for a few minutes for the anaesthetic to take effect. Sometimes objects get under the third eyelid, so look carefully at the edge of it.

2 Remove the object.

With your finger and thumb, or with tweezers, carefully pick up the object and remove it from the eye. Make sure the animal's head is held firmly.

3 Flush the eye.

With clean, boiled water, squirt the surface of the eye using a syringe without a needle.

4 Ointment.

If the surface of the eye is scratched, use ointment as described in the next section.

16.4 Damage to the surface of the eye

The surface of the eye, called the cornea, can be damaged by straw or twigs and other things that get into the eyes, or by accidents where the surface of the eye is hit.

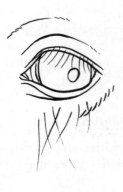

What damage to the surface of the eye looks like
- The surface of the eye may be grey-white instead of clear.
- A small crater may be seen on the glassy surface of the eye.
- The eye is watering more than usual.
- The animal may keep the eye closed.
- If infected, there may be yellow-white discharge around the eyes.

- Later on, when a deeper injury is healing, a small blood vessel grows across the surface of the eye as the damage heals.

How to prevent injury to the surface of the eye

See the note about fitting blinkers (blinders) properly in the section *The healthy eye.*

How to treat injuries to the surface of the eye

Prevent infection with eye ointment containing antibiotic (such as oxytetracycline, neomycin, chloramphenicol). See the list of ointments at the back of the book. See the next section for how to use it.

Do not use ointment containing corticosteroid (such as prednisolone, betamethasone) because these drugs slow down the rate of healing.

16.5 Infection around the eyes, conjunctivitis

What conjunctivitis looks like

- Reddened skin inside the eyelids.
- More tears and usually a sticky, yellow discharge around the eyes.

How to prevent conjunctivitis

- Control flies, which carry infection to the eyes.
- A fly fringe is useful to keep flies out of the eyes.
- If horses' or donkeys' eyes are affected by dust, bathe around the eyes with clean cloth or cotton wool soaked in warm, boiled water. Use new, clean cotton wool for each animal, or you may take infection from one animal to the next on the cotton wool.
- If one animal has eye infection, wash your hands after treating it, before touching other horses.

How to treat conjunctivitis

Apply antibiotic eye ointment. Follow the manufacturer's instructions. Usually it is recommended that ointment is applied three or four times per day (because the tears wash medication out of the eye) and that the treatment is continued for five days.

With the thumb of one hand, roll down the lower eyelid. With the base of your other hand against the horse's head (so that if it moves its head, your hand moves with it and the end of the tube does not go into its eye), squeeze ointment along the inside of the lower eyelid.

16.6 Periodic ophthalmia, moon blindness

This is the commonest form of blindness of horses and follows a particular type of infection around the eyes. This infection comes and goes, eventually leading to damage to the eyesight. It is also called recurrent uveitis.

What periodic ophthalmia looks like
- Usually one is eye affected, but both may be involved.
- More tears from the affected eye.
- The eyelids stay partly closed.
- There is pain in the eye.
- The animal does not like bright light.
- The skin inside the eyelids is red.
- The glassy surface of the eye may be grey at the edge.

At a late stage, without treatment, the eye becomes greyish-white and shrunken. There is no effective treatment at this stage.

How to prevent periodic ophthalmia
Follow the same advice as for prevention of conjunctivitis.

How to treat periodic ophthalmia
- Keep the horse in a darkened place.
- Treat with an eye ointment containing corticosteroids (see list at back of book). Continue the treatment for four weeks.

Even with treatment, it is possible that the animal will become blind.

16.7 Growths (tumours)

Tumours sometimes grow around the eyes in older horses. The only treatment is surgical. A veterinary surgeon must deal with these cases.

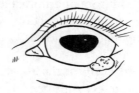

16.8 Eyelid turning in

Some foals are born with eyelids that turn in, usually only the lower lids. The eyelashes then rub on the surface of the eyes, causing soreness and tears.

How to treat in-turned eyelids of foals
- Inject local anaesthetic into the skin where the stitching needle will go in.
- Stitch together two folds of skin below the lower eyelid to stretch the skin and roll the eyelid out.

16.9 Blocked and swollen tear ducts

This condition commonly affects donkeys in some places, such as parts of Egypt. Some vets say that it is related to epizootic lymphangitis (see the section *Epizootic lymphangitis, pseudoglanders*), but it responds to treatment for worms, just like habronemiasis (see the section *Summer sores, habronemiasis*). Therefore, small worms are probably the cause.

What tear duct infection looks like

- Tears roll down the cheek on the affected side.
- Hair is lost below the inside corner of the eye.
- There may be swellings below the eye.

How to treat tear duct infection

1 Treat with ivermectin (see the section *Summer sores, habronemiasis*).
2 Give antibiotic injections, for example, penicillin with streptomycin.
3 Give eye ointment containing antibiotic and corticosteroid (for examples see the list at the back of the book).
4 Trained people may flush the blocked tear duct with boiled, warm water (or salt solution used for intravenous drip). The debris is flushed up the tear duct from the nose.

Call vet!

Advanced cases have raw skin down the face from the inside corners of the eyes.

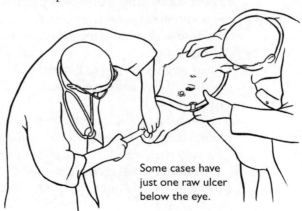

Some cases have just one raw ulcer below the eye.

- If a metal needle is used it must have a rounded end. Alternatively, a flexible plastic catheter can be used.
- The needle or catheter is attached to a 20 ml syringe containing boiled, warm water (or saline from a bag for intravenous drip).
- The needle or catheter is put in the opening of the tear duct in the nostril and water is squirted up the duct.
- When the blockage is cleared, water will be seen streaming out of the inside corner of the eye.

17 Poisoning

17.1 About poisons and general treatment

Some poisons cause sudden death. Others cause a wide range of signs, depending on which parts of the body are damaged.

Many poisons have an unpleasant taste and are avoided by animals. Thin, hungry animals are more likely to eat poisonous substances.

How to treat poisoning

Some poisons have a particular treatment, described below. If you do not know exactly what the poison was, use these general treatments.

TREATMENT TO ADSORB THE POISON

- Give **charcoal** by mouth or stomach tube (see the section *How to use a stomach tube*). Many poisons 'stick' (adsorb) to charcoal and so less poison gets into the body. Activated charcoal adsorbs best and is available from pharmacies. Charcoal made from animal bones is very good for adsorbing poison. Any charcoal has some benefit but, if using wood charcoal, grind it and make sure there are no small sticks in the mixture.
- The dose of charcoal depends on the body weight of the animal. Mix the ground-up charcoal in water, about 200 g charcoal per litre of water. Give 500 g charcoal in 2.5 litres water to a horse that weighs 400 kg. (The dose of charcoal is 1–3 g per kg body weight of the animal.)
- The charcoal can be mixed with **milk** instead of water. Milk is helpful for poisons that irritate the lining of the guts.
- As an alternative to charcoal, give **kaolin**. The disadvantage of kaolin is that it will reduce diarrhoea, which is nature's way of getting the poison out of the body. Kaolin suspension is available as a human medicine from pharmacies. Give about 200 ml of this liquid by mouth.

TREATMENT TO MAKE THE POISON GO THROUGH THE BODY FASTER

- Give a treatment to make the animal pass dung. For example, **liquid paraffin** (*not* fuel paraffin/kerosene) or **castor oil**. This is best given by stomach tube (see the section *How to use a stomach tube*), but can be given from a bottle, taking care that the animal swallows the fluid and does not choke on it.

- Kaolin or charcoal can be given mixed with liquid paraffin.
- **Magnesium sulphate** (**Epsom salts**) is also effective in speeding the passage of the poison through the guts. The dose for a horse is 200–300 g dissolved in 4 litres of warm water. (Smaller animals need less, according to their body weight.) It is best given by stomach tube. Charcoal can be given in the same mixture, without increasing the quantity of water.

TREATMENT TO REDUCE DAMAGE TO THE INSIDE OF THE GUTS

- For poisons that irritate the lining of the guts, give a **mixture of eggs, sugar and milk**. For an adult horse give 3 eggs and 50 g of sugar mixed with 250 ml milk. Repeat with the same again after 30 minutes.

17.2   Poisonous plants

There are so many different chemicals in different plants that many different effects on animals may be seen. Most animals avoid eating poisonous plants. Some poisonous plants are more likely to be eaten if cut and dried with grass for hay.

Examples of plant poisoning

What the poisoning looks like	Examples of poisonous plants
• Colic and diarrhoea	• Acorns, *Ranunculus* species (e.g. buttercup)
• Colic, diarrhoea and strange behaviour	• *Belladonna* species (nightshade), hemlock
• Weakness, strange walking and falling over (see below for more information)	• Bracken ferns (*Pteridium* species) or horsetail (*Equisetum* species) eaten for a month or more
• Sudden death	• Yew tree (*Taxus*), sorghum
• Photosensitization (see the section *Sunburn, photosensitization*)	• *Senecio* species (e.g. ragwort), *Hypericum* species (e.g. St John's wort)
• Stiff walking, swelling around the roots of the teeth (secondary hyperparathyroidism)	• Some tropical pasture grasses (e.g. *Setaria* species, guinea grass or *Panicum maximum*)

17.3   Bracken and horsetail plant poisoning

Bracken (*Pteridium* spp.) and horsetail (*Equisetum* spp.) are both poisonous plants, but horses need to eat a lot for several weeks to develop signs of poisoning.

What bracken or horsetail poisoning looks like
- Weakness and staggering,
- trembling muscles,
- eventually the animal may lie down with its neck stretched out and die.

How to treat bracken or horsetail poisoning
Inject vitamins, making sure that the mix contains thiamine, vitamin B_1.

17.4 Lead poisoning

Young horses are affected more than older ones. Slowly developing lead poisoning is more common than sudden, severe poisoning.

What lead poisoning looks like
- Weakness,
- difficulty breathing in and snoring sounds,
- drooling saliva,
- sometimes difficulty swallowing and food may come back down nose,
- sometimes lung infection (pneumonia),
- may stagger around, appearing blind.

How to avoid lead poisoning
- Give enough food to reduce the animal's desire to eat strange things.
- Do not paint fences or the inside of buildings with paint containing lead.

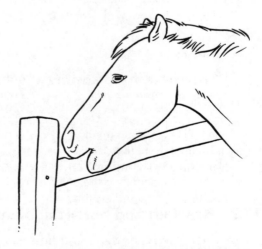

- Do not leave old car batteries where animals graze.
- Do not let animals graze near factories where lead is processed.

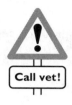

Call vet!

How to treat lead poisoning

The treatment for lead poisoning is calcium versanate (another name for this is calcium disodium ethylenediamine tetra-acetate or EDTA), dose 75 mg per kg body weight. The amount calculated for the body weight is given over a three-day period, preferably by drip into the vein (a veterinarian will be needed to set this up). Mix calcium versanate with saline so there is 20 mg of calcium versanate per litre (2% solution) in the drip solution. After four days, repeat the treatment.

17.5 Organophosphate poisoning

Some sprays and dips contain organophosphates, which are used to kill insects and ticks. These chemicals are used to treat animals and are also common as plant sprays.

What organophosphate poisoning looks like
- Muscle twitches and nervous appearance,
- sweating and diarrhoea.
- The centre, black part (pupil) of the eye becomes a narrow slit.
- If severe the animal may develop fits.
- Unlike other animals, organophosphate poisoning does not usually make horses drool.

How to treat organophosphate poisoning

Give atropine injection slowly (over several minutes) into the vein, dose around 1 mg per kg body weight (the exact amount needed depends on how much poison is in the body).

Observe the effect on the animal as you give it. If you are in a shady place and the centre, black part of the eye becomes bigger, stop giving the atropine. It may be necessary to repeat the treatment after about five hours.

17.6 Ivermectin poisoning

Horses may become ill if ivermectin (Ivomec) injection for cattle is used. If ivermectin for cattle is injected into the muscle of the horse, sometimes these signs occur:

- Swelling where the injection was given,
- swelling (oedema) of the belly,
- swelling of legs and eyelids,
- difficulty breathing,
- colic,
- sudden death.

17.7 Mouldy food

Some types of fungi that grow on animal food produce poisonous substances.

What disease from mouldy food can look like
- Dull behaviour,
- loss of appetite,
- trembling,
- staggering,
- lying down,
- death.

There is no treatment. Prevent this kind of poisoning by storing food dry and not giving mouldy feed to animals.

17.8 Botulism

Botulism is a rare type of paralysis. It is usually caused by accidentally eating the poison in decayed meat; grazing animals can get botulism if a rat or mouse has died in a haystack or if water birds have died in a lake where the animals drink.

What botulism looks like
- Trembling muscles and sweating,
- weakness of the legs and stumbling,
- weakness of face muscles gives a sleepy expression,
- after a few days the animal goes down and lies on its side,
- breathing is difficult,
- the animal usually dies.

How to prevent botulism
- Dispose of dead bodies hygienically.
- In the USA vaccine is sometimes given to mares during pregnancy to protect foals.

Treatment
There is no widely available, effective treatment.

17.9 Snake bite

What a snake bite looks like
The signs depend on which type of snake bit the horse or donkey.

- Painful swelling that appears quickly,
- muscle twitching,
- widening of the pupil (the black part in the centre of the eye),
- sweating,
- weakness.

How to treat a snake bite
- If the bite is on a leg, put a tourniquet above the bite. To do this, take a strip of cloth and tie it into a loop around the leg. Put a

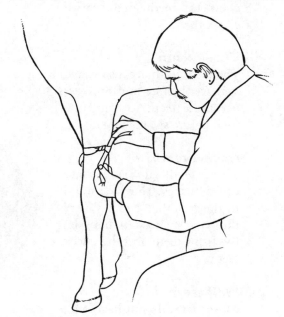

piece of stick in the loop and twist it until the loop becomes tight around the leg. Every 20 minutes, loosen the loop for a few minutes. Continue for several hours.
- Snake bites often become infected. Therefore, give antibiotic injections.
- Check whether the animal is vaccinated against tetanus. If not give tetanus antitoxin (see the section *Tetanus*).
- If help is available from an expert who knows about the snakes in the area and has appropriate antidotes, give an injection of antivenin as quickly as possible.

18 Teeth and how to tell the age

18.1 Horse and donkey teeth

Horses' and donkeys' teeth keep growing during their lives. As the animals graze and chew, the teeth wear against each other.

Cheek teeth

The back teeth are also called 'molars'. Horses and donkeys use these teeth to grind the food before swallowing it.

Canine teeth

These teeth are sometimes called 'tushes'. They are found in the mouths of males, very rarely in mares, in between the front teeth and the cheek teeth.

Wolf teeth

Most mares do not have 'wolf teeth'. If present in the mouths of males, they grow just in front of the top row of cheek teeth.

Some people believe that wolf teeth cause problems, such as interfering with the bit. Therefore, sometimes they are removed, usually when the animal is two or three years old. Other experts do not believe that wolf teeth really interfere with the bit, which lies across the bottom

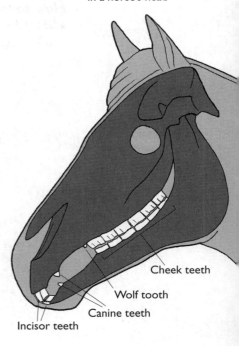

The position of teeth in a horse's head

Cheek teeth

Wolf tooth

Canine teeth

Incisor teeth

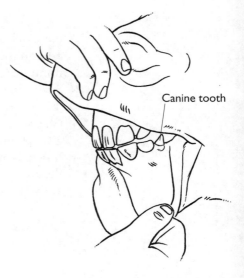

Canine tooth

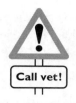

jaw, and so they do not recommend that they be removed.

This is a job for an experienced person, who may use a special extractor tool for the job.

Front teeth

The front teeth are also called 'incisors'. They are used to bite and pluck the grass when an animal is grazing.

There are three pairs of front teeth. The middle front teeth are called 'centrals'. The outside ones are called 'corners'.

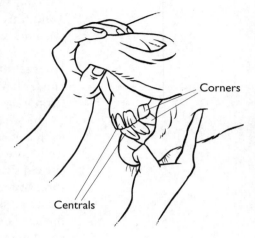

18.2 How to tell the age of a horse or donkey by its teeth

Horses may live to 40 years old and donkeys to more than 50 years. You can estimate the ages of younger horses and donkeys by looking at the changes in growth and wear of the upper and lower front teeth. Ageing horses is difficult at first, but becomes easier with practice.

Like us, horses and donkeys first grow a set of temporary or 'baby' teeth, and later adult teeth. Unlike us, horses' and donkeys' teeth keep growing during their lives and their teeth wear down as they eat.

We work out the age, first, by which of the front teeth have grown. Later, we estimate the age by how much the front teeth have worn down.

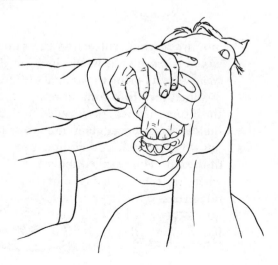

Using the teeth to tell the age up to 4½ years old is accurate. Above this age, the teeth give a guide, but the changes are less accurate indicators of the animal's age.

Horses and ponies

Horses have six top and six bottom front teeth. Foals grow all the temporary set of front teeth in their first year of life.

The adult teeth come up later. The middle (central) pair of adult teeth appears when the animal is 2½ years old. The next adult front teeth grow through when 3½ and 4½ years old. Look for the difference in size of the big adult and small temporary teeth at the age of three or four years.

At five years old, the animal has all its adult teeth. In the next years the age is estimated by the wear of the front teeth. This shows as changing patterns on the biting surface of these teeth. The pattern changes because the tooth is not the same inside all the way down. Therefore, the biting end looks different as the tooth wears down.

If we were to remove a whole front (incisor) tooth from the head of a young horse, it would look like this:

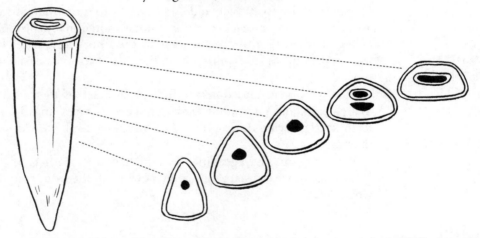

If we were to cut across the same tooth in different places, it would show how it would look on the biting surface as the tooth wears down during the animal's life.

When they first come through, the front teeth have a hollow in the biting surface. This is called the 'cup'. As the horse gets older, this hollow gets more circular and grows to the back of the tooth, and is known as a 'mark'. A dark line is seen on the biting surface, in front of the cup. This is called the 'star'.

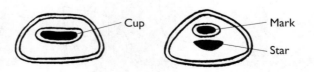

Cup

Mark

Star

Later, the mark grows out and only the star is left on the biting surface.

Telling the age of horses and ponies by the appearance of the teeth

Age of horse or pony	What the front or side of the teeth look like	Appearance of biting surface of front teeth	Description
Three years old			First pair of adult teeth has grown and is in wear.
Four years old			Second pair of adult teeth is up and in wear. One pair of baby teeth is left.
Five years old			Third (corner) pair of adult teeth is up and is wearing down at the front.
Six years old			The teeth have worn level and all have a central indent called a 'cup'. The corner teeth are now wearing level.
Seven years old			The cup is less deep in the central pair of front teeth, where it is now called a 'mark'. There is still a good cup in the other front teeth. At seven years, a 'hook' can be seen on the side of the upper corner front teeth.

The seven-year hook

Age of horse or pony	What the front or side of the teeth look like	Appearance of biting surface of front teeth	Description
Eight years old			A dark line at the front of the teeth (called a 'star') has appeared on each of the central pair of front teeth.
Nine years old			Now no more cups, only marks. Stars have appeared on the next teeth. A groove begins to grow down the upper corner front tooth.

The groove that appears at nine years old

Ten years old			The biting surfaces are more triangular. The star has appeared on the corner front teeth. Stars are becoming more round and nearer the middle of the tooth. Marks are less distinct. The 7 year hook has worn away.
12 years old			The mark has gone from the centrals. Stars are now round. The groove in the upper corner teeth is about 1 cm long.
15 years old			Only stars on the teeth. The groove is now half way down the upper corner teeth.
19–20 years old			Seen from the side, the teeth have a forward slope. The groove extends down the whole tooth.

Age of horse or pony	What the front or side of the teeth look like	Appearance of biting surface of front teeth	Description
20–25 years old			The teeth have an even more forward-pointing angle and the groove is growing out (it disappears at about 30 years old). The tops of the teeth now have a more triangular shape.

Donkeys

Donkeys also have six top and six bottom front teeth. Ageing by growth of new front teeth is similar to horses. New adult incisors appear at 2½, 3½ and 4½ years old. Ageing donkeys up to five years old is done in the same as horses. After that there are some differences:

- Donkeys' corner front teeth may not be fully in wear until nine or ten years old (compare the horse – six years old).
- The cups can still be seen in some donkeys' lower front teeth until around 20 years old. In horses, the cups disappear by ten years old.
- The groove, which occurs from nine years of age in horses' upper corner front teeth, does not appear in donkeys. Also the hook on the same tooth which is seen in horses is not a reliable guide for ageing donkeys.

18.3 Tooth rasping

The back teeth of some horses and donkeys do not wear evenly. Sharp edges can develop on the cheek teeth and can stop the animal eating properly.

A good policy with all horses and donkeys more than 15 years old is to rasp the teeth once or twice per year. It is worth inspecting the cheek teeth of all animals more than ten years old, and rasping them if necessary every few months.

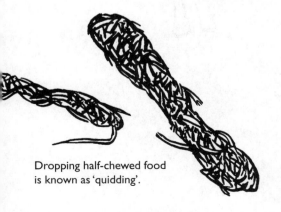

Dropping half-chewed food is known as 'quidding'.

What tooth problems look like

Suspect tooth problems if the animal chews for some time and spits out its mouthful.

Suspect tooth problems if an older horse is thin. A horse with poor teeth does not eat properly.

How to rasp (or 'float') teeth

The tool used is a kind of file on a handle. Ideally, for upper teeth, a rasp with a bend in the handle is used, and for lower teeth a straight one is used.

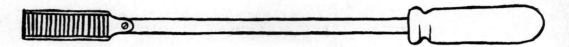

The sharp edges develop on the *outside* of the *top* rows of cheek teeth and on the *inside* (the side nearer the tongue) of the *bottom* cheek teeth. So the rasp is angled to smooth down these edges of the rows of teeth.

An assistant holds the horse's head. The person doing the rasping normally grasps the horse's tongue and rasps the sharp edges of the teeth.

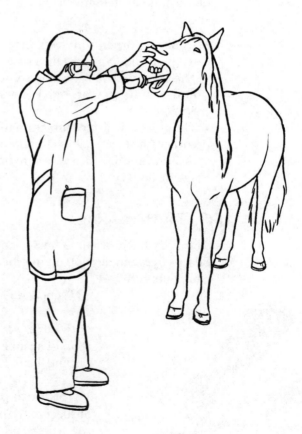

19 Heat stress

In hot climates, working horses and donkeys may become over-heated especially in the hot season. If the over-heating is severe, the animal may die.

What heat stress looks like
- Panting or laboured breathing,
- wide open nostrils,
- droopy, lowered head,
- dull behaviour,
- high heart rate,
- increased body temperature,
- less elastic skin.

To see if the skin is less elastic, pinch a fold of skin on the neck. Normally, the pinched up skin will lie flat again almost straight away. If the horse is dehydrated, the skin stays pinched up for some time.

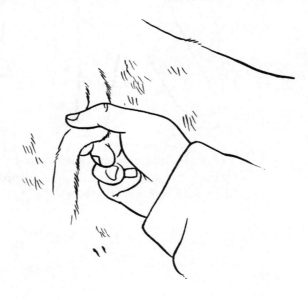

How to prevent heat stress

- In hot weather, offer water to working horses and donkeys at least four times per day. *Little and often* is the best rule for drinking water.
- Give a hot animal enough time at the drinking place. If it is hot, a horse or donkey may need at least five minutes before it is ready to drink.
- Find a shady place for working animals to stand in the heat of the day.

How to treat heat stress

Pour buckets of water over the animal's back. Rub the water into its hair to wet the skin.

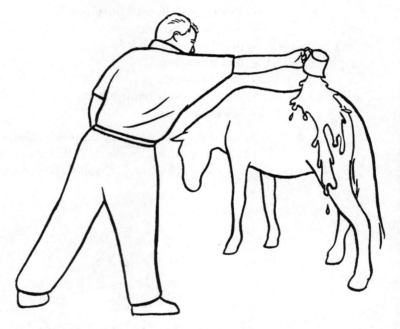

Stand it in the shade. Offer a bucket of water to drink and let the animal rest until its breathing is normal (see the section *Temperature, heart rate and breathing*).

20 How to shoot a horse

The two humane methods used to kill horses are lethal injection and shooting. The drugs used for lethal injections are only available to veterinary surgeons. This section explains how to shoot a horse or donkey.

Guns are dangerous. Therefore:

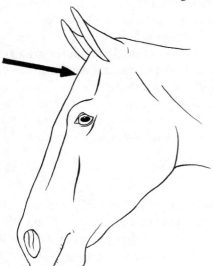

- Obey laws about gun ownership and using guns.
- Do not shoot if people are standing around the horse.
- Do not shoot a horse near a wall or a hard road in case the bullet bounces off and kills or injures someone.
- Be sure anyone helping you stands behind you when you fire the gun.

Where to put the end of the gun

Imagine lines between the middle of the eyes and the middle of the base of the ears. The end of the gun is positioned above the point where the lines cross.

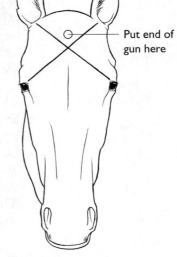

Put end of gun here

Angle of aim

Aim the gun as shown in the picture.

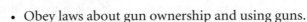

What happens when the shot is fired

If you fire the shot as instructed, the bullet goes through the brain. The horse immediately falls down. Its body will be still, but the legs may move around for a short time. The hole where the bullet went in will bleed and blood may come out of the nose.

Medicines

Information about medicines

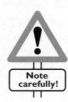

Medicines and the law

- In most places, according to the law, only qualified veterinarians should buy most of the drugs in the lists below, and, by law, people who are not vets should only use them on animals that are under a veterinarian's care. You should be aware that, if you buy and use these medicines and you are not a registered veterinarian, you may be breaking the law.
- If you use a medicine in a way that is not included in the manufacturer's instructions, even if that way is described in this book, it is your own responsibility.
- Such a use might be giving to a horse or donkey a medicine that has not been registered for use with horses or donkeys. If the animal health worker or owner decides to use that medicine on a horse or donkey, he or she must accept the risk.
- Although every effort has been made to ensure that the advice in the lists of medicines is safe and accurate, no responsibility can be accepted for any problem arising.

Storing medicines

- Store medicines in a place where children cannot reach them.
- Do not keep half-used medicines in food or drink bottles, unless they are labelled and kept locked up.
- Most medicines should be stored in a cool place, but not frozen.
- Whenever possible, use medicines before the expiry date.
- If medicines have been stored cool, most are effective and can be safely used for some time after the expiry date stated on the label.
- A few medicines must be stored in a refrigerator. Follow the manufacturer's instructions.

Names of medicines

- The 'Examples of manufacturer's product names' given in the lists below are mainly taken from products available in the UK. Drug companies marketing in other countries may use different names for the same products. Check the 'Drug name' column to see whether products with other product names contain the same things.

- New products with new names are being released all the time.

How to give medicines

- Always follow the manufacturer's warnings and instructions.
- Carefully read the data sheet, which should always be included with a new package of medicine.
- See the chapter *How to give medicines* for the method for giving injections and other ways to give medicines.
- In that chapter, see the section *How to work out the amount of medicine to give* for an explanation of working out how much to give.

Local remedies, medicinal plants, 'ethnoveterinary medicine' and local healers

- In all societies, there is knowledge of traditional medicine. Often this involves using medicinal plants that grow locally. Many of these treatments are effective and their use has clear advantages. For example, they are always available and they are cheap or free.
- Local healers have useful knowledge. It is wise to consult them and ask for their advice.
- Local remedies are not discussed in detail in this book, partly because many of them are used only in the places where particular medicinal plants grow, and so are not relevant all over the world. However, that does not mean that this book does not recommend their use.
- In this book, 'firing' or burning the skin with hot irons is discouraged. There is no scientific evidence that branding is an effective treatment. It causes unnecessary suffering to the animal.

Lists of medicines mentioned in the book

1   Medicines for treating infections
2   Medicines for treating pain, inflammation and allergy
3   Medicines for killing worms and stomach bots
4   Medicines for treating colic
5   Medicines for treating wounds
6   Medicines for maggots in wounds (fly-blown wounds)
7   Medicines for treating skin diseases and for killing parasites on the skin
8   Medicines for preventing diseases
9   Medicines for eye diseases
10 Medicines for treating poisoning
11 Medicines for sedating animals
12 Other medicines

u

Drugs in this group are mainly antibiotics. Antibiotics are effective against infections caused by bacteria.

Drug type	Drug name	Examples of manufacturer's product name	Examples of what it is used for	How much to give	How to give it	How many times per day to give it	How long to give it	Notes and warnings
Antibiotic	penicillin long-acting injection (mix containing 150 mg procaine penicillin and 112.5 mg benzathine penicillin in each ml)	Depopen-P, Duphapen LA, Duplocillin LA, Lentrax 100, Norocillin LA, Penillin LA, Procillin LA, Propen, Vetipen	Infection in the foot with fever, infected wound with fever, tetanus, anthrax	8 ml per 200 kg body weight	IM injection	1	Give one injection only	This mixture of penicillin is 'long-acting'. Normally, only one injection is necessary.
Antibiotic	penicillin (300 mg procaine penicillin per ml or 300 000 IU per ml)	Depocillin	Dermatophilosis, kidney and bladder infections, ulcerative lymphangitis. It can also be used for the conditions listed under long-acting penicillin injection.	12 mg per kg body weight (for 200 kg animal, give 8 ml)	IM injection	1	3–5 days	This kind of penicillin needs to be given once per day. Under different product names (such as Duphapen, Econopen, Lenticillin, Norocillin, Penillin) the same kind of penicillin is recommended by the manufacturers for use in cattle, sheep and pigs, but may not be registered for horses.

I Medicines for treating infections (cont.)

Drug type	Drug name	Examples of manufacturer's product name	Examples of what it is used for	How much to give	How to give it	How many times per day to give it	How long to give it	Notes and warnings
Broad-spectrum antibiotic	penicillin with streptomycin (each ml contains 200 mg procaine penicillin and 250 mg dihydro-streptomycin sulphate)	Depomycin Forte, Duphapen+Strep, Penicillin/ Streptomycin Injection, Pen and Strep, Streptopen Injection	Infection in the foot with fever, swollen joint with fever, infected joints, cuts and injuries involving tendons or joints, infectious diseases affecting breathing, sinusitis, diarrhoea caused by an infection, retained placenta with fever, mastitis, blocked and swollen tear ducts	8 mg penicillin and 10 mg streptomycin per kg body weight (8 ml per 200 kg body weight) – the strength of the mix varies between manufacturers, so check the instructions	IM injection	1	3 days Infections of joints and tendons may need more days treatment. Sinusitis may need 2–3 weeks treatment. For delay as soon as it is decided that there may be infection in the joint.	Under different product names (such as Dipen Forte, Penillin PS, Strypen Injection) penicillin and streptomycin is recommended by manufacturers for cattle, sheep and pigs.
Antibiotic	penicillin with gentamicin	Pangram (gentamicin only)	Joint-ill of foals	Follow manufacturer's instructions on dose of gentamicin	IM injection	1	7–10 days	Gentamicin products may not be licensed for use in horses and donkeys.
Broad-spectrum antibiotic	ampicillin injection (each ml contains 150 mg ampicillin)	Amfipen, Duphacillin, Norobrittin, Penbritin	Diarrhoea caused by an infection	7.5 mg per kg body weight (for a product with 15% ampicillin, i.e. 150 mg per ml, give 10 ml to a 200 kg animal)	IM injection	1	3–5 days	

1 Medicines for treating infections (cont.)

Drug type	Drug name	Examples of manufacturer's product name	Examples of what it is used for	How much to give	How to give it	How many times per day to give it	How long to give it	Notes and warnings
Broad-spectrum antibiotic	ampicillin powder	Amfipen	Proud flesh	Break open eight 250 mg capsules and mix the powder with 50 ml boiled and cooled water	Wash the wound	1 or 2	7 days	These capsules are commonly sold as human medicine.
Antibiotic	metronidazole injection (each ml contains 450 mg metronidazole)	Torgyl	Canker, thrush, infected hoof wounds	If using 45% solution (that is, 450 mg metronidazole per ml), give 10 ml to a 200 kg animal.	IM injection. If used on a dressing, replace after 48 hours	1	2–5 days	A weak solution can be used on dressings applied to the infected area or squirted on to wounds to wash them.
Broad-spectrum antibiotic	oxytetracycline	Engemycin, Tetcin, Terramycin	Canker	Enough to soak a pad of cotton wool or cloth	Bandage the pad on to the infected part	1	Until healthy, maybe months	The named formulations of the drug are sold for injecting cattle, sheep and goats. If stressed horses or donkeys are injected with oxytetracycline it may cause severe diarrhoea.

1 Medicines for treating infections (cont.)

Drug type	Drug name	Examples of manufacturer's product name	Examples of what it is used for	How much to give	How to give it	How many times per day to give it	How long to give it	Notes and warnings
Broad-spectrum antibiotic	potentiated sulphonamides (each ml contains 40 mg trimethoprim and 200 mg sulphadiazine or sulphadoxine, but see note about Tribrissen 48%)	Delvoprim Coject, Duphatrim IS, Norodine 24, Trimabac Injection 24%, Trivetrin Injection, Tribrissen Injection 48%	Diarrhoea caused by an infection, liver disease, kidney and bladder infections, mastitis, epizootic lymphangitis, glanders	15 mg of combined ingredients per kg body weight (15 ml injection for 240 kg body weight)	Slowly inject into a vein (but give Tribrissen 48% by IM injection). Sulphonamides are also available to give to horses by mouth as powder or pre-filled paste syringes.	1	Up to 5 days	The mix of ingredients in Tribrissen Injection 48% is double the strength of the others listed, and, therefore, half the volume is needed for the same body weight of animal. Tribrissen 48% is given by IM injection.
Antiserum	tetanus antitoxin	Tetanus Antitoxin (sometimes 1000 IU per ml, but sometimes other concentrations)	To prevent tetanus in animals not vaccinated against tetanus after wounds, such as nail in the foot. To treat tetanus	When treating wounds, give 3000 IU for a foal or small horse or donkey and 5000 IU for a larger animal. When treating tetanus, give 50 000–150 000 IU	When treating wounds, IM or SC injection. When treating tetanus, inject slowly into a vein	1	One dose to prevent tetanus	If treating tetanus, inject daily for 1 week.
Antiseptic	copper sulphate	Copper sulphate	Thrush	50 g crystals in 1 litre water	Wash infected area	1 or 2	Until infection has disappeared	

I Medicines for treating infections (cont.)

Drug type	Drug name	Examples of manufacturer's product name	Examples of what it is used for	How much to give	How to give it	How many times per day to give it	How long to give it	Notes and warnings
Antiseptic or disinfectant	formalin	Formalin	Thrush, canker	To make 1 litre solution, add 50 ml formalin to 950 ml water	Wash infected area	1 or 2	Until infection has disappeared	Wear plastic or rubber gloves when mixing the solution. Mix outside, not in a room with closed windows.
Antiseptic	potassium permanganate	Potassium permanganate	Thrush	Dissolve crystals to give a strong purple colour	Wash infected area	1 or 2	Until infection has disappeared	
Trypanosome killer	homidium bromide	Ethidium, Novidium	African trypanosomiasis	1–2 mg per kg body weight	IM injection	1		
Trypanosome killer	quinapyramine sulphate	Antrycide, Trypacide, Noroquin	African trypanosomiasis	2.2–4.4 mg per kg body weight	SC injection. There may be a painful reaction at the place where the injection is given. To reduce the reaction, split the dose between two or three parts and inject in different places.	1		There are problems of resistance to this drug, which means it is no longer always effective against African trypanosomiasis.

I Medicines for treating infections (cont.)

Drug type	Drug name	Examples of manufacturer's product name	Examples of what it is used for	How much to give	How to give it	How many times per day to give it	How long to give it	Notes and warnings
Trypanosome killer	quinapyramine sulphate	Antrycide, Trypacide, Noroquin, Quintrycide	Surra	3 mg per kg	SC injection	Work out total dose, give half in first injection	Give the other half in a second injection six hours later	There may be a painful reaction at the place where the injection is given. Rub or massage the place after giving the injection.
Trypanosome killer	diminazine aceturate	Berenil	Surra	7 mg per kg body weight	IM injection	24 hours after first injection, give a second injection of half the dose of the first one		Toxic to horses, but sometimes used.
Trypanosome killer	diminazine aceturate	Berenil	African trypanosomiasis	3.5 mg per kg body weight	IM injection	1		Toxic to horses, but sometimes used.
Trypanosome killer	isometamidium chloride	Trypamidium, Samorin	Surra	0.5 mg per kg body weight	IM injection	1		See the section *Surra* for advice on dilution. Split the total dose, and inject into two or three places. Rub or massage the place after giving the injection.
Babesia killer	imidocarb dipropionate 12%	Imidocarb	Babesiosis	2 ml per 100 kg body weight	IM injection	1	A second injection may be needed after 48 hours	There are two species of the *Babesia* parasite that affect horses. One species, *B. cabelli*, is normally treated with one injection. The other species, *B. equi*, may need the second injection after 48 hours for successful treatment.

2 Medicines for treating pain, inflammation and allergy

This group contains corticosteroids and NSAIDs (non-steroidal anti-inflammatory drugs). Do not use NSAIDs in an animal that may have kidney disease. Do not use corticosteroids in an animal that may have an infection or laminitis.

Drug type	Drug name	Examples of manufacturer's product name	Examples of what it is used for	How much to give	How to give it	How many times per day to give it	How long to give it	Notes and warnings
NSAID	phenylbutazone	Equipalazone, Pro-Dynam	Old arthritis with new bone around the joint, ring bone, side bone, bony spavin, splints, sore shins, navicular disease, bog spavin, thoroughpin	2.2 mg phenylbutazone per kg body weight (half of one 1 g sachet of powder to an animal weighing 225 kg)	By mouth, mixed with some tasty food	Every second day	Treatment can be continued for a long time for old animals with arthritis	Available as powder and as paste. Reduce the dose to the minimum amount necessary to keep the animal comfortable. Stop using if there is no improvement after 5 days treatment. Not recommended for animals with kidney disease.
Corticosteroid	betamethasone injection (2 mg betamethasone per ml)	Betsolan Injection	Allergic reaction, purpura, blocked and swollen tear ducts	5–20 ml depending on size of animal	IM injection	1	One injection is usually sufficient	Do not use in pregnant animals. Can cause laminitis. Corticosteroids slow wound healing.
Corticosteroid	dexamethasone injection (2 mg dexamethasone per ml)	Colvasone, Dectan, Dexadreson, Dexazone, Duphacort Q, Soludex, Voren	Allergic reaction, purpura, blocked and swollen tear ducts	1 ml per 50kg body weight	IM injection	1	One injection is usually sufficient. If continued treatment is needed, give the injection as advised by manufacturer (usually 1–2 weeks after first injection).	Do not use in pregnant animals. Corticosteroids slow wound healing.

2 Medicines for treating pain, inflammation and allergy (cont.)

Drug type	Drug name	Examples of manufacturer's product name	Examples of what it is used for	How much to give	How to give it	How many times per day to give it	How long to give it	Notes and warnings
Corticosteroid	dexamethasone (2 mg per ml) injection	As above	Viral encephalitis	0.05–0.1 mg per kg body weight (5–10 ml for a 200 kg animal)	IM injection	Give every 6–12 hours	2 days	Do not use in pregnant animals. Corticosteroids slow wound healing.
NSAID	flunixin meglamine 50 mg per ml	Finadyne Solution	Colic, viral encephalitis, cut tendon	For colic or injury, 1 ml per 45 kg body weight (5 ml for 225 kg body weight animal). For encephalitis, 0.5 mg per kg body weight (5 ml per 200 kg body weight)	IV injection for colic. IM injection if IV not possible in horse with encephalitis	Once for colic. Every 12 hours for encephalitis	One injection may be enough for colic. For other conditions, give for several days as necessary	Finadyne is also available as medicine to give by mouth. Do not give to an animal with kidney disease.
NSAID	ibuprofen	Brufen	Old arthritis	1.5–2 g for an adult horse; 1 g is four 250 mg tablets	Grind tablets and mix with treacle or tasty food	1	As necessary	The tablets are a human medicine.
Corticosteroid	prednisolone	Prednisolone tablets	Purpura, allergic reaction, chronic pulmonary disease (CPD), old arthritis and other long-term conditions, new bone around the joint	For purpura, 5 mg prednisolone per 10 kg body weight. For arthritis and other long-term conditions, give the minimum dose that keeps the animal comfortable	Grind tablets and mix with tasty food	2	As necessary	Corticosteroids slow wound healing.
Bee sting remedy	sodium bicarbonate	Baking soda	Bee stings	Mix a tablespoonful with 100 ml water	Soak a piece of cloth or cotton wool and apply to the stings	Treat as soon as possible after the animal is stung		

3 Medicines for killing worms and stomach bots

Drug type	Drug name	Examples of manufacturer's product name	Examples of what it is used for	How much to give	How to give it	How many times per day to give it	How long to give it	Notes and warnings
Worm killer	mebendazole	Equivurm, Telmin	Gut roundworms	5–10 mg mebendazole per kg body weight	By mouth	1	Usually, at least 6 weeks between treatments	Give according to need and worming programme (see the chapter *Diarrhoea, worms and other parasites living inside the body*).
Worm killer	oxibendazole	Equidin	Gut roundworms	10 mg oxibendazole per kg body weight (but 15 mg oxibendazole for young foals with diarrhoea)	By mouth	1	Usually, at least 6 weeks between treatments	Give according to need and worming programme (see the chapter *Diarrhoea, worms and other parasites living inside the body*).
Worm killer	fenbendazole	Panacur	Gut roundworms	7.5 mg fenbendazole per kg body weight. Fenbendazole can be given as a single dose at higher dose rates: for migrating red-worm larvae, give 60 mg per kg body weight; for treating diarrhoea of young foals, give 50 mg per kg body weight	Mix liquid suspension or granules with tasty food. Squirt paste directly into the mouth	1	Daily for 5 days (but one dose on one day only at higher dose rates)	Give according to need and worming programme (see the chapter *Diarrhoea, worms and other parasites living inside the body*).

3 Medicines for killing worms and stomach bots (cont.)

Drug type	Drug name	Examples of manufacturer's product name	Examples of what it is used for	How much to give	How to give it	How many times per day to give it	How long to give it	Notes and warnings
Parasiticide	ivermectin	Eqvalan paste, Furexel paste, Panomec paste	Stomach bots, gut roundworms	0.2 mg per kg body weight	By mouth	1		In countries with a cold winter, the best time to treat for bots is early winter. See notes on using ivermectin injection in the list *Medicines for maggots in wounds*.
Worm killer	pyrantel	Strongid-P, Pyratape P	Tapeworms, gut roundworms	For tapeworms give double dose of 38 mg per kg. For roundworms give 19 mg per kg	If powder, mix with food. If paste, give directly into mouth	1	If treatment for tapeworm is necessary, dose can be repeated every 6 weeks	Treatment for tapeworm is not usually necessary.
Parasiticide	ivermectin	Eqvalan paste, Furexel paste, Panomec paste	Lung worms	0.2 mg per kg body weight	By mouth	1	One treatment only	See notes on using ivermectin injection in the list *Medicines for maggots in wounds*.
Worm killer	mebendazole	Equivurm, Telmin	Lung worms	For donkeys, give 15–20 mg per kg (for a 200 kg donkey, give up to 10 g of granules containing 100 mg per gram)	If granules, mix with food. If paste, give directly into mouth	1	5 days	

3 Medicines for killing worms and stomach bots (cont.)

Drug type	Drug name	Examples of manufacturer's product name	Examples of what it is used for	How much to give	How to give it	How many times per day to give it	How long to give it	Notes and warnings
Worm killer	fenbendazole	Panacur	Lung worms	15 mg per kg body weight	If liquid suspension or granules, mix with tasty food. If paste, squirt directly into mouth	1	One treatment	
Worm killer	thiabendazole	Thibenzole	Lung worms	440 mg per kg body weight and repeat after 2 days		1	Repeat after 2 days	
Fluke killer	triclabendazole	Fasinex	Liver fluke	It is suggested to use maker's recommended dose rate for cattle	By mouth			This medicine is sold for cattle.

4 Medicines for treating colic

Drug type	Drug name	Examples of manufacturer's product name	Examples of what it is used for	How much to give	How to give it	How many times per day to give it	How long to give it	Notes and warnings
Spasm reducer and pain reliever	4 mg hyoscine with 500 mg dipyrone per ml	Buscopan Compositum	Spasmodic colic, choke (food stuck in neck)	20–30 ml (less if a very small horse or donkey)	IV injection	1	One injection is usually enough	The colic pain should disappear quickly after injection if the colic is caused by gut muscle spasm.
NSAID	flunixin meglamine 50 mg per ml	Finadyne Solution	Spasmodic colic	1 ml per 45 kg body weight (5 ml for 225 kg body weight animal)	IV injection	1	One injection may be enough for colic	Can be repeated after 24 hours.
NSAID	phenylbutazone 200 mg per ml	Equipalazone Injection	Gas colic	Up to 4.4 mg per kg body weight. Maximum 5 ml for animal of 225 kg body weight	IV injection given slowly	1	One injection should be enough	
NSAID	flunixin meglamine 50 mg per ml	Finadyne	Gas colic	1.1 mg per kg body weight (or 5 ml for 225 kg body weight animal)	IV injection	1	One injection may be enough for colic	Can be repeated after 24 hours.
Laxative	liquid paraffin	Liquid paraffin	Impaction colic	2–4 litres	By mouth, preferably by stomach tube	2	3 days	Liquid paraffin is *not* the same as paraffin (kerosene) fuel.

5 Medicines for treating wounds

Drug type	Drug name	Examples of manufacturer's product name	Examples of what it is used for	How much to give	How to give it	How many times per day to give it	How long to give it	Notes and warnings
Local anaesthetic	lignocaine 2% (sometimes with adrenaline)	Locaine, Lignocaine, Lignavet	Stitching cuts	0.5 ml at each place	Subcutaneous injection about 10 minutes before stitching		It lasts for 30 minutes (or can last longer if adrenaline is included in the mix)	Before injecting, try to suck back with syringe plunger: if blood is drawn back into the syringe, do not inject in that place.
Mild antiseptic	povidone-iodine	Betadine, Pevidine, Pyodine	Cleaning fresh wounds	Make a very dilute solution using plenty of water	See the section *How to care for a fresh wound*	2	Until healing is advanced	Do not use povidone-iodine made for washing hands because this contains detergent that could harm the wound.
Antibacterial spray	'purple spray' (usually contains a tetracycline with gentian violet or marker dye)	Alamycin Aerosol, Duphacycline Aerosol, Ocyretin Aerosol, Tetcin Aerosol	Wounds on the hoof	Enough to cover infected place	Spray on to affected area	1	Daily as necessary	It is better to wash skin wounds with mild antiseptic, rather than use an aerosol spray. The products listed may be registered only for sheep or for cattle, sheep and pigs.
Healing ointment	zinc oxide ointment	To make 1 kg of this ointment, add 150 g zinc oxide powder to 850 g petroleum jelly (Vaseline) and mix well	Cracked heels	Enough to thinly cover the wound	Apply to wound	1	Repeat every few days until healed	Some olive oil can be added into the mix.

5 Medicines for treating wounds (cont.)

Drug type	Drug name	Examples of manufacturer's product name	Examples of what it is used for	How much to give	How to give it	How many times per day to give it	How long to give it	Notes and warnings
Ointment	petroleum jelly	Boroline, Vaseline	Pressure sores, burns, cracked heels, on gauze for wound dressing, to lubricate a thermometer or stomach tube	Enough to make a thin layer	Apply to affected area	1 or 2	Daily or as necessary	
Ointment containing corticosteroid	May contain betamethasone, prednisolone, triamcinolone	Betsolan Cream, Dermobion Ointment (registered for use in horses), Vetalog Plus Cream	Proud flesh only	Just enough to cover the proud flesh	Apply to the proud flesh, but *not* to the edges of healthy skin around it	2	Continue until proud flesh is smaller	Never use corticosteroid ointment on any other type of wound. Not all the products listed are registered for horses.
Antiseptic	iodine	Tincture of iodine	Infected wounds, epizootic lymphangitis	Add to clean water to make a light brown solution (the colour of weak black tea)	See the section *How to care for a fresh wound*			
Antiseptic	mercurochrome		Infected wounds	Add a pinch of crystals to water to make a red solution	See the section *How to care for a fresh wound*			

5 Medicines for treating wounds (cont.)

Drug type	Drug name	Examples of manufacturer's product name	Examples of what it is used for	How much to give	How to give it	How many times per day to give it	How long to give it	Notes and warnings
Antibiotic ointment	(various)		Infected wounds	Cover wound with a thin layer	Apply to infected wound	1 or 2	Daily as necessary	Antibiotic ointment is commonly available as a human medicine. Ointments made for treating mastitis in cattle have been used on infected wounds.
Soothing lotion	calamine		Burns	Pour lotion on to cotton wool or clean cloth	Apply gently to the burnt skin	2	Until healing is progressing well	
Antiserum	tetanus antitoxin	Tetanus Antitoxin (sometimes 1000IU per ml, but sometimes other concentrations)	Any deep or dirty wound, snake bite	3000IU for a foal or small horse or donkey and 5000IU for a larger animal	IM or SC injection	1	One dose	

6 Medicines for maggots in wounds (fly-blown wounds)

Most of the medicines for killing parasites on the skin (like ticks, lice and flies) are effective against maggots.

Drug type	Drug name	Examples of manufacturer's product name	Examples of what it is used for	How much to give	How to give it	How many times per day to give it	How long to give it	Notes and warnings
Maggot killer	coumaphos with propoxur (and sulphanilimide)	Negasunt	Maggots in wounds	Enough to cover wound	Clean the wound. Sprinkle the powder on the wound and the surrounding skin	1	Repeat after 24 hours if there are live maggots in the wounds	Wash hands carefully after using. Poisonous for fish, so do not contaminate water.
Maggot killer	boric acid powder with turpentine oil (or with kerosene)	Mix the powder with the oil (or kerosene) to make a thick paste	Maggots in wounds	Enough to cover wound	Apply direct to wound	1	One application should be sufficient	
Maggot killer	chloroform		Maggots in wounds	Soak cotton wool or clean cloth	Hold on the wound	2	Until there are no more live maggots	Be careful not to breathe the fumes. Use outdoors, not inside with closed windows.

6 Medicines for maggots in wounds (cont.)

Drug type	Drug name	Examples of manufacturer's product name	Examples of what it is used for	How much to give	How to give it	How many times per day to give it	How long to give it	Notes and warnings
Parasiticide	ivermectin	Ivomec 1% injection (for cattle), Eqvalan paste, Furexel paste, Panomec paste	Maggots in wounds	If it is given by mouth the dose is 0.2 mg per kg body weight (40 mg for 200 kg body weight of horse, that is, 4 ml of 1% solution for injection). If using paste syringe, follow manufacturer's dose instructions	By mouth. 2 or 3 drops of solution for injection can be placed directly on to the wound	1	One dose only	Putting it directly on the wound is not a use recommended by the manufacturer, but has been seen to rapidly kill maggots. The form sold as cattle injection has been given to horses by mouth, after mixing it with tasty food or just squirting it directly into the mouth. Ivermectin injection for cattle can cause poisoning (see the chapter *Poisoning*) to horses if injected. Dangerous for fish, so do not contaminate water even with empty container.
Pour-on pyrethroid acaricide	deltamethrin or flumethrin	Spot-On or Bayticol	Maggots in wounds	A few ml	Pour on to maggoty area	1	One treatment should be sufficient	May not have been tested on horses. Dangerous for fish, so do not contaminate water even with empty container.

7 Medicines for treating skin diseases and for killing parasites on the skin

Medicines containing pyrethroids or ivermectin are poisonous for fish. Take care not to dispose of unused medicine or even the empty containers in rivers or ponds.

Drug type	Drug name	Examples of manufacturer's product name	Examples of what it is used for	How much to give	How to give it	How many times per day to give it	How long to give it	Notes and warnings
Insect repellent	pyrethrum and piperonyl butoxide, or permethrin and citronellol	Sweet Itch Lotion, Lincoln Sweet Itch Control, Coopers Fly Repellent Plus for Horses	Sweet itch	Give enough to reach the skin at the base of the hair of the mane and tail. Follow manufacturer's instructions	Part the hair and apply to skin of the mane, back and tail with a brush or cloth	1	Every day during fly season	Placing the horse under a roof from mid-afternoon reduces attack by the flies (Culicoides) that cause sweet itch. This product is dangerous to fish.
Insect repellent, insecticide	4% permethrin	Switch, Beatitch	Sweet itch	10 ml per 100 kg body weight up to a maximum dose of 40 ml	Pour on to mane and rump. Avoid saddle area	1	Weekly in the season	Dangerous for fish.
Insect repellent, insecticide	5% cypermethrin concentrate	Deosan Deosect	Control of flies (including Culicoides, Stomoxys, Haematobia, tabanids, tsetse, mosquitoes), sweet itch, lice	125 ml of diluted solution per animal (more if a large horse)	Dilute with water (20 ml concentrate in 1 litre of water). Spray on to skin	1	Repeat after 1 month in the fly season. Can be repeated after 1 or 2 weeks if fly problem is severe. For lice control, repeat after 2 weeks	Dangerous for fish.
Organo-phosphorus acaricide (tick and mite killer)	coumaphos	Asuntol	Ticks, mange, harvest mites	Dilute with water according to manufacturer's instructions	As a spray	1	No more than once per week	Take care not to get organophosphorus compounds on your skin. Wear plastic or rubber gloves.

7 Medicines for treating skin diseases (cont.)

Drug type	Drug name	Examples of manufacturer's product name	Examples of what it is used for	How much to give	How to give it	How many times per day to give it	How long to give it	Notes and warnings
Pour-on pyrethroid acaricide	deltamethrin or flumethrin	Spot-On or Bayticol Pour-on	Ticks, mange mites, harvest mites	10 ml per 100 kg body weight, but check manufacturer's instructions	Pour on to the back	1	Repeat after 2 weeks if necessary	May not have been tested on horses, so use at your own risk. Dangerous for fish.
Parasiticide (worm, tick and mite killer)	ivermectin paste	Eqvalan paste, Furexel paste, Panomec paste	Mange mites, summer sores/ bursatti, some lice	0.2 mg per kg body weight	By mouth	1	One treatment should be sufficient	Not effective against chewing lice like *Damalinia*. See notes on using ivermectin injection in the list *Medicines for maggots in wounds*.
Insecticide powder	permethrin, for example	Louse Powder (Arnolds)	Lice, rubbing post against flies	For lice treatment, about 50 g	Shake powder from shoulders along the back to the rump	1	Lice usually need 2 or 3 treatments with an interval of 10 days	Dangerous to fish.
Insecticide	piperonyl butoxide and pyrethrum	Dermoline shampoo	Lice	Mix 100 ml of shampoo in 1 litre of water. Use at least 1 litre per horse	Pour the diluted shampoo on to the back of the animal. Add more shampoo and use a brush to get a good lather	1	Repeat after 10–14 days	Do not get into the animal's eyes. Wear rubber or plastic gloves when applying it.

7 Medicines for treating skin diseases (cont.)

Drug type	Drug name	Examples of manufacturer's product name	Examples of what it is used for	How much to give	How to give it	How many times per day to give it	How long to give it	Notes and warnings
Antifungal agent	griseofulvin	Equifulvin, Fulcin, Grisol-V, Grisovin, Norofulvin	Ringworm	10 mg per kg body weight	If granules or powder, mix with tasty food. If paste, give by mouth	1	Daily for 7 days. In severe cases, continue for 1 more week	Do not use in pregnant animals. It should not be handled by pregnant women nor by women of child-bearing age unless wearing plastic gloves.
Disinfectant	chlorhexidine 4%	Hibiscrub, Savlon (also contains cetrimide)	Ringworm	Mix 25 ml (or 10 ml of Savlon) in 1 litre of water	With a sponge or cloth, apply to ringworm	1 or 2	For several weeks until ringworm has gone	Wash hands carefully with soap after touching ringworm.
Disinfectant	sodium hypochlorite solution	Clorox	Ringworm	Mix 100 ml of Clorox in 1 litre of water	With a sponge or cloth, apply to ringworm	1 or 2	For several weeks until ringworm has gone	Wash hands carefully with soap after touching ringworm.
Antibiotic ointment	Various, for example containing penicillin or tetracyclines		Dermatophilosis	Enough to cover the affected skin	Apply after carefully removing scabs	1	Until the skin has healed	Antibiotic ointment is often sold for use on human wounds.
Antibiotic	penicillin	See the list *Medicines for treating infections*	Dermatophilosis	As for other infections, see the list *Medicines for treating infections*	IM injection	1	5 days	
Antiseptic	iodine	Tincture of iodine	Ulcerative lymphangitis, epizootic lymphangitis	Dilute with water to give the colour of weak, black tea	Use it to wash the lesions and to flush them by squirting it into burst abscesses	1	Daily until lesions have healed	

8 Medicines for preventing diseases

Drug type	Drug name	Examples of manufacturer's product name	Examples of what it is used for	How much to give	How to give it	How many times per day to give it	How long to give it	Notes and warnings
Vaccine	tetanus toxoid	Duvaxyn T, Tetanus Toxoid Concentrated	Prevent tetanus	1 ml	SC or IM injection	Give once and repeat 1 month later	Booster injections every few years maintain good immunity	Give foal its first injection when more than 3 months old. Manufacturer may recommend more frequent boosting. If tetanus antiserum has been given, wait 4 weeks before vaccinating. Tetanus and flu vaccines are available together in a combined vaccine.
Vaccine	killed or inactivated strains of flu virus	Duvaxyn IE, Prevac	Prevent flu	1 ml	IM injection	Give once and repeat after 1 month. Inject again after 6 months	Give a booster injection every 2 years	Give first injection to foal when at least 2 months old. If the first injection is given when less than 6 months old, repeat when 6 months old.
Vaccine	inactivated strain of rabies	Nobivac Rabies	Prevent rabies	1 ml	IM injection	Give once and repeat 1 month later	Give a booster injection each year	Not recommended for pregnant mares.
Vaccine	For North America, contains strains of EEE and WEE. For South America, may contain VEE as well		Prevent viral encephalitis		IM injection	Give once and repeat 1 month later. It is usually given in spring, 1 month before the mosquito season	Give a booster injection each year. In high risk areas, boosters may be given every 3 months	Give first injection to foal when it is more than 3 months old. Boost vaccination before the season when mosquitoes that carry the virus are common.

9 Medicines for eye diseases

Drug type	Drug name	Examples of manufacturer's product name	Examples of what it is used for	How much to give	How to give it	How many times per day to give it	How long to give it	Notes and warnings
Antibiotic eye ointment	tetracycline eye ointment	Aureomycin Ophthalmic Ointment	Conjunctivitis	About 5 cm squirted directly from the tube	Apply ointment across the inside of the lower eyelid and gently massage	3	Until eye appears normal, up to 5 days	
Antibiotic eye ointment	chloramphenicol eye ointment	Chloromycetin Ophthalmic Ointment	Conjunctivitis	About 5 cm squirted directly from the tube	Apply ointment across the inside of the lower eyelid and gently massage	3	Until eye appears normal, up to 5 days	
Antibiotic eye ointment	neomycin eye ointment	Neobiotic Eye Ointment	Conjunctivitis	About 5 cm squirted directly from the tube	Apply ointment across the inside of the lower eyelid and gently massage	3	Until eye appears normal, up to 5 days	
Antibiotic eye ointment	cloxacillin eye ointment	Orbenin Ophthalmic Ointment, Kloxerate	Conjunctivitis	About 5 cm squirted directly from the tube	Apply ointment across the inside of the lower eyelid and gently massage	1	Repeat once per day	Sometimes only one single treatment with this ointment is needed.
Corticosteroid eye drops	betamethasone (may also contain neomycin antibiotic)	Betsolan Eye Drops, Neobiotic HC Drops	Periodic ophthalmia	2 drops per eye	Hold the upper eyelid up and drop medicine on to surface of eye	4	Repeat daily as necessary	Never use eye medicine with corticosteroid if the eye is injured, for example, an eye with an ulcer.
Antibiotic plus corticosteroid eye ointment	chloramphenicol with hydrocortisone	Choloromycetin Hydrocortisone Ointment	Blocked and swollen tear ducts	A few cm squirted directly from the tube	Apply ointment across the inside of the lower eyelid and gently massage	4	Repeat daily as necessary	Never use eye medicine with corticosteroid if the eye is injured, for example, with ulcer.

10 Medicines for treating poisoning

Drug type	Drug name	Examples of manufacturer's product name	Examples of what it is used for	How much to give	How to give it	How many times per day to give it	How long to give it	Notes and warnings
Adsorbant	activated charcoal		General treatment for poisoning	1–3 kg depending on the animal's body weight	Mix with water to make a slurry and give by mouth	1	1 day	Take care it does not cause choking when swallowed. Stomach tube recommended.
Adsorbant	kaolin suspension		General treatment for poisoning	About 100 ml for a donkey; and 200 ml for an adult horse	By mouth	1	Once should be sufficient	Kaolin reduces diarrhoea, but diarrhoea may be useful to get poison out.
Laxative	liquid paraffin		General treatment for poisoning	2–4 litres	By mouth, preferably by stomach tube	1	Once should be sufficient	Helps speed the passage of the poison by making the animal pass dung.
Laxative	castor oil		General treatment for poisoning	1–2 litres	By mouth, preferably by stomach tube	1	Once should be sufficient	Helps speed the passage of the poison by making the animal pass dung.
Purgative	magnesium sulphate	Epsom salts	General treatment for poisoning	200–300 g dissolved in 4 litres of warm water	By mouth, preferably by stomach tube	1	Once should be sufficient	Helps speed the passage of the poison by making the animal pass dung.

10 Medicines for treating poisoning (cont.)

Drug type	Drug name	Examples of manufacturer's product name	Examples of what it is used for	How much to give	How to give it	How many times per day to give it	How long to give it	Notes and warnings
Antidote	calcium disodium ethylenediamine tetra-acetate or calcium versanate	EDTA	Lead poisoning	75 mg per kg body weight	Add 20 mg calcium versanate per litre of saline drip and give IV as a drip	Once	Repeat dose after 4 days	A trained person should set up and monitor the drip.
Antidote	atropine sulphate 0.6 mg per ml	Atrocare Injection, Atropine Sulphate Injection	Organo-phosphorus poisoning	Depends on how much poison is in the body. Dose approximately 0.1–0.2 mg per kg body weight (33–66 ml for a 200 kg animal)	Slow IV injection of one quarter of the dose. SC injection of the remainder of the dose	Once, if the signs of poisoning are relieved. Injection may be repeated after 4 hours if signs of poisoning come back		Do not give more than 10 ml SC injection at one place to a donkey, or 15 ml SC to a horse.

11 Medicines for sedating animals

Drug type	Drug name	Examples of manufacturer's product name	Examples of what it is used for	How much to give	How to give it	How many times per day to give it	How long to give it	Notes and warnings
Sedative	acetyl promazine 10 mg per ml	ACP Injection	Tetanus	Up to 0.1 mg per kg body weight (2 ml for a 200 kg animal). Response varies, so if half this dose is sufficient to sedate the horse, give reduced dose	IM injection or slow IV injection	1	Repeat every 36–48 hours to control signs of tetanus	Can cause problems in stallions, causing the penis to come out of its sheath and not go back. If this happens, it may be necessary to quickly anaesthetize or cast the animal and reduce the penis swelling by squeezing it or by bandaging it.
Sedative	diazepam	Diazemuls, Diazepam, Valium	Viral encephalitis	For a foal weighing 50 kg, 5–20 mg. For an adult animal weighing 200 kg, give 10–40 mg	Slow IV injection	Repeat if fits start again	1 day	This drug is licensed for use in people. Smaller doses may be effective. Give as much as needed to stop fits.
Sedative	xylazine 100 mg per ml	Chanazine 10%, Rompun, Virbaxyl 10%	Viral encephalitis	For a foal weighing 50 kg, inject 25–50 mg, that is 0.25–0.5 ml. For an adult animal weighing 200 kg, give 1.0–2.0 ml. If fits are severe a higher dose may be needed	Slow IV injection	Repeat if fits start again	1 day	Do not disturb the animal in the first 5 minutes while the medicine takes effect. Effects are seen after about 5 minutes and last for about 20 minutes, but animals stay drowsy for several hours. Do not use in the last month of pregnancy.

12 Other medicines

Drug type	Drug name	Examples of manufacturer's product name	Examples of what it is used for	How much to give	How to give it	How many times per day to give it	How long to give it	Notes and warnings
Multivitamin	Vitamin injection including B vitamins	Anivit, Combivit, Duphafral Extravite, Multivet 4BC, Multivitamin Injection (Arnolds)	Liver disease, plant poisoning with bracken or *Equisetum*	Depends on concentration in the product. Follow manufacturer's instructions	IM injection or slowly by IV injection	1	It depends on the disease. The injection can be repeated as necessary	
Hormone	oxytocin injection (10 IU per ml)	Hyposton, Oxytocin Leo, Oxytocin-S, Pituitary Extract (Synthetic)	Retained placentas, difficult birth (but only on the advice of a vet)	1–4 ml	Slowly by IV injection. Can be given IM	1	One dose is normally enough	It is best if a trained person gives it using a drip.
Water soluble gel	lubricant gel, obstetric lubricant	KY Jelly, Vet-lube	To make the hands and arms slippery when helping with a difficult birth	Smear it on your hands and arms and then rub a little water with it to make it more slippery				
Mineral	calcium borogluconate solution 20%	Calcibor, Calciject, CBG-20, Calc no. 1, Rycal no. 1	Hypocalcaemia	Dose varies. About 500 ml is required for an adult horse	Slowly by IV injection		Normally once is enough for recovery	May cause heart problems if given too fast. A trained person should give it. These products are not usually registered for horses.

Index